For Thomas and Yvonne Eaton, purveyors of fine moral compasses and unconditional love, encouragement and support.

Contents

About the Authors

Aidan Baron is a paramedic researcher and educator from Sydney, Australia. His main interests are paramedic point of care ultrasound, evidence-based practice education, applied ethics and patient advocacy. He has been a visiting researcher in emergency, cardiovascular and critical care at Kingston University and St George's, University of London in the UK, and also a member of faculty in the discipline of paramedicine at Charles Sturt University, Australia.

Edd Bartlett is a paramedic with an interest in mental capacity, mental health and human rights. After completing a BSc (Hons) in Paramedic Practitioner (Community Emergency Health) at the University of Plymouth, he went on to gain an MA in Medical Ethics and Law at King's College London. Alongside this, he worked full time as a paramedic at the South East Coast Ambulance Service, before being seconded onto its Frequent Caller Team. Moving away from full time employment in the ambulance service, he then worked as a Court of Protection and mental health paralegal at Bison Solicitors before taking up his current position as Legal Services Manager for Surrey and Borders Partnership NHS Foundation Trust. Edd is also a visiting lecturer for paramedic education at Birmingham City University. He supports reform of the Mental Capacity Act 2005 and the Mental Health Act 1983, moving towards a 'fusion' approach and compliance with the United Nations Convention on the Rights of Persons with Disabilities. Edd is grateful to dissertation tutors, Professor Penney Lewis and Alison Ross from King's College London, for their guidance and support during his Master's, from which his chapter on Mental Capacity draws. He would also like to thank Dr Gareth Clegg, Dr Matthew Reed and Mr Gabriel Oniscu for sharing the Royal Infirmary of Edinburgh Maastricht Category II Donation after Circulatory Death procedures and their correspondence in the writing of Chapter 13.

Keiran Bellis is Lecturer in Paramedic Science at the School of Health Sciences at the University of Central Lancashire. Within this role, he is responsible for overseeing the delivery of all the ethical and legal aspects of paramedic practice education and interprofessional learning within the Paramedic Science programme. With undergraduate degrees in law and psychology, his research interests lie with pre-hospital ethics, mental capacity and suicide. Having previously been employed as an associate lecturer at the Lancashire Law School, he has been involved in a number of EU-funded research projects and has lectured globally on many topics, including law and ethics, bioethics and paramedic practice. He joined the Greater Manchester Ambulance Service in 2000 prior to moving to Lancashire in 2003 before the services merged to create the North West Ambulance Service in 2006. Still an operational paramedic, he combines academia with frontline duties in both the private and NHS sectors. He is also a peer reviewer for the *Journal of Paramedic Practice* and *Studies in Ethics, Law, and Technology*, and has published in the *Journal of Interprofessional Care*.

Will Broughton is a paramedic and senior lecturer in Paramedic Science at the University of Hertfordshire. He has a BSc (Hons) in Paramedic Science from the University of Hertfordshire and an MSc in Paediatrics and Child Health from Imperial College London. He continues to practise as a paramedic in the London and South Central regions of the UK. He is the Director of Professional Standards for the College of Paramedics. He is also an active expert witness and has a special interest in developing paediatric education for paramedics as well as improving the clinical outcomes for children attended by frontline clinicians. He is supporting a national project led by the Royal College of Paediatrics and Child Health to develop a national paediatric early warning score for use in the UK. He is a peer reviewer for the *British Paramedic Journal* and the *Emergency Medicine Journal*. He was editor-in-chief for the UK version of the *Advanced Medical Life Support* and *Prehospital Trauma Life Support* courses textbook and has authored two chapters for the *Paediatric Education for Prehospital Professionals* course textbook.

Vince Clarke works at the University of Hertfordshire, where he has been employed since 2016. He joined the London Ambulance Service in 1996, qualified as a paramedic in 1998 and entered the Education and Development Department in 2001. He worked as part of the Higher Education Team and developed in-house paramedic programmes as well as working closely with higher education partner institutions. A Health & Care Professions Council partner since 2006, he has been involved in the approval of a wide range of paramedic educational programmes across the country, as well as assessing Continuing Professional Development submissions and sitting on Conduct and Competence Fitness to Practise panel hearings. He works closely with the College of Paramedics, sitting on the Education Advisory Committee and undertaking the role of Head of Endorsements. He also works as an independent paramedic expert witness for the Courts and prepares reports on breach of duty for both claimants and defendants.

Andy Collen is the Medicines and Prescribing Project Lead for the College of Paramedics, working alongside NHS England mainly on independent prescribing for advanced paramedics, as well as other projects such as the review of paramedic medicines exemptions. He is responsible for the College's published documents relating to medicines and has prepared practice guidance for prescribers, and implementation guidance for prescribing, as well as practice guidance for exemptions. He is currently a consultant paramedic at the South East Coast Ambulance Service and leads the Trust's specialist/advanced paramedic practice programmes, professional standards and scope of practice. He is also the author of *Decision Making in Paramedic Practice* and has contributed to a range of other titles, including one on development about different aspects of medicines in paramedic practice.

Georgette Eaton is an Advanced Paramedic in Primary and Urgent Care. Trust. Prior to this appointment, she split her employment between clinical practice and education, balancing work as a specialist paramedic in urgent care across a range of settings with being Senior Lecturer in Paramedic Science at Oxford Brookes University. Alongside this, she has been the regional South Central Trustee for the College of Paramedics (2017–19) and continues to be a member of the Education Advisory Group and the Primary and Urgent Care Special Interest Group within the professional body.

She was a graduate paramedic from Coventry University in 2011 and after 'topping up' to BSc (Hons) began practising as a specialist paramedic (then an emergency care practitioner). She completed her first MSc in Critical Care at Cardiff University in 2017 and her second in Education Research Design and Methodology at the University of Oxford in 2018. She is currently reading for a DPhil in Evidence-Based Healthcare at the Nuffield Department of Primary Health Care, University of Oxford.

Samantha McCabe-Hogan is a senior lecturer at Sheffield Hallam University, lecturing in theoretical subjects such as research, law, ethics and public health. Before joining the ambulance service, she was in the Royal Air Force and worked at her local hospital as a nursing assistant. She joined the Lincolnshire Ambulance Service in 2001 in Health Transport and moved into Emergency Operations in 2003, qualifying as a paramedic in 2006. As well as working on the front line, she worked in both the education and research departments at the East Midlands Ambulance Service. Her undergraduate degree is in Health Studies (2003) and her Master's is in Clinical Research (2009).

Tom Mallinson was drawn to the bright (blue) lights of the big city and started his medical career as a paramedic and Chemical Biological Radiation and Nuclear (CBRN) operative for the London Ambulance Service NHS Trust. He then decided to read Medicine at the University of Warwick, before gaining further qualifications in healthcare education and pre-hospital medicine – subjects for which he remains a passionate advocate as an active researcher in the field. Not content to trade the action of the ambulance service in completely, he has since built a career that combines research with response, working as a flight doctor in the Bailiwick of Jersey, and in both anaesthesia and critical care in the Midlands. He has more recently migrated north, working as a GP and voluntary responder for the Scottish Ambulance Service with the support of BASICS Scotland and the Sandpiper Trust. Now based in the wilds of the Outer Hebrides, he is able to also practise his other passion of wilderness medicine through volunteering for the Hebrides Mountain Rescue Team and HM Coastguard. In spite of all of this adventure, he has always said that the part of his career that has resonated most with him was his time working with the palliative care team on Jersey, training under Dr Nicky Bailhache, who remains a big inspiration. This proved to be a formative experience, balancing the dedication stemming from his paramedic training to do everything possible in the moment with the need for compassion and respect for a patient's individual needs. He hopes the reader finds his thoughts on the matter both interesting and helpful.

John Renshaw is Senior Lecturer in Paramedic Science at Coventry University and a part-time PhD student at Kingston University and St George's, University of London. He first graduated with a foundation degree in Paramedic Science in 2011 and subsequently worked as a Paramedic and Clinical Team mentor for the West Midlands Ambulance Service NHS Foundation Trust. He then studied for a BSc (Hons) in Pre-hospital and Emergency Care, a postgraduate certificate in Academic Practice in Higher Education, and joined the paramedic team as a senior lecturer in 2016. Alongside this role, he is an editorial board member for the *Journal of Paramedic Practice*, an Adult Advanced Life Support Instructor for the Resuscitation Council (UK), and a student member of the Emergency, Cardiovascular and Critical Care Research group at Kingston University and St George's, University of London.

Ceri Sudron is Senior Lecturer and BSc Course Lead for Paramedic Science at the University of Wolverhampton. She began her career as a paramedic with the West Midlands Ambulance Service, progressing to paramedic clinical mentor with South Central Ambulance Service in 2007 and later as a Clinical Education Development Specialist with the East Midlands Ambulance Service. In 2015, she joined the University of Northampton's paramedic teaching team before returning full circle to the Midlands and the University of Wolverhampton. She completed her MSc in Practice Education in 2014 and focused on the leadership of professional practice, culminating in a dissertation exploring the professional identity of the paramedic and the identification of professional attitudes and behaviour. Her research interests include CPR-induced consciousness, professionalism, organisational culture, LGBT+ health inequality, education and mentoring. She is an editorial board member and an active reviewer for the *Journal of Paramedic Practice*.

Note from the Editor

I am incredibly proud of the contributory author team within this book. The book is unique in two aspects: first, all authors are paramedics (including Dr Mallinson, who is dual registered as a GP and paramedic). Second, all authors have specialised (clinically, within education, leadership or research) in the areas in which they write about. In 2019, we are at a point in the development of the profession that paramedics are not only writing their own text books but they are also specialising in subjects relevant to the profession. It is an incredibly exciting time to be a paramedic, and if you are joining the profession now, then the world really is your proverbial oyster. Each of these authors give their voice to comment on how their issue relates to paramedic practice and, regardless of your stage in practice, I am confident this book has something for everyone – from student through to consultant. As you read through these chapters, think about you. Take pride in your professional title and know what it means. Continue to look, listen and learn – from your patients, your peers and your supervisors. Think about who *you* are, what values you hold dear to you and where you sit within the world. Remember the legal boundaries that govern your practice. But above all, *enjoy* it. There is no job in the world that is more rewarding than being the person who is called upon to help humanity at its worst. . . and by your very presence allows humanity to act its best. Regardless of your clinical setting, regardless of wherever you sit within clinical practice, education, leadership or research, of all the healthcare professionals, we are the most privileged. Never let go of that.

Chapter 1

Introduction

Georgette Eaton

Contemporary healthcare is complex. Since the National Health Service (NHS) was established in 1948, the three initial core principles have expanded, with seven principles that underpin the modern healthcare system. Evolving from the financial themes of the 1940s, today's core principles focus on access to services, quality of care received and patient safety.

Then and Now: The Core Principles of the NHS (Department of Health 2015)

The NHS was created with the ideal that good healthcare should be available to all, regardless of wealth. On 5 July 1948, Aneurin Bevan (Minister for Health) outlined three core principles to underpin the NHS:

- That it meets the needs of everyone.
- That it be free at the point of delivery.
- That it be based on clinical need, not the ability to pay.

In October 2015, the Department of Health updated the NHS Constitution for England, which sets out the guiding values of the NHS and the evolution of the initial concepts to seven core principles:

- The NHS provides a comprehensive service available to all.
- Access to NHS services is based on clinical need, not an individual's ability to pay.
- The NHS aspires to the highest standards of excellence and professionalism.
- The NHS aspires to put patients at the heart of everything it does.
- The NHS works across organisational boundaries and in partnership with other organisations in the interests of patients, local communities and the wider population.
- The NHS is committed to providing best value for taxpayers' money and the most effective, fair and sustainable use of finite resources.
- The NHS is accountable to the public, communities and patients that it serves.

Over the last 70 years, the NHS has seen an unprecedented rise in demand across its services (Wankhade 2010), a situation that has been compounded by a reduction in funding and a population which has a greater awareness of their rights and services as patients. Within this change is encapsulated the ambulance service and the role of the paramedic. The paramedic profession has evolved considerably since its inception some 20 years after the founding of the NHS (Collen 2017) and with many NHS ambulance services now positioned as mobile healthcare providers, the paramedic role has consequently evolved. Paramedics increasingly provide clinical assessment and management, using a variety of delivery methods both remotely (using a hear-and-treat approach) or face to face (using a see-and-treat or see-and-refer model) (NICE 2017). Paramedics are no longer confined to four wheels and the modern paramedic has the opportunity to practise in diverse clinical areas, such as acute hospital trusts, forensic healthcare, primary care practices, critical care services, minor injury units and urgent care centres (Evans et al. 2013; Williams et al. 2013; O'Meara 2014). Paramedics are also not limited to clinical practice, with an emerging presence within the academy as well as research. Leadership posts across a range of NHS and private services also boast paramedics. The changing demands on the ambulance service have birthed a twenty-first-century paramedic who is expected to be nothing if not a generalist (Eaton et al., 2018).

A key driver of the transformation of paramedics in care provision has been their level of autonomy as allied health professionals. Unlike other parts of the world, UK paramedics are required to register with the Health and Care Professionals Council (HCPC). Registration changed many aspects of paramedic practice, with the professional standards becoming central to professional practice and underpinning patient care. It also ensured that paramedics became accountable for their actions and, whilst this is discussed in more detail in Chapter 2, it is worth noting that this accountability reflects the professional identity of the profession. As well as ensuring that the modern paramedic acts competently, this registration also outlines ethical standards that paramedics must comply with in order to ensure both quality of care and patient safety.

Quality of Care

The quality of care provided by healthcare organisations is overseen by different bodies in England, Northern Ireland, Scotland and Wales.

England

Established as part of the National Health Service Act 2006, the Care Quality Commission (CQC) and Monitor regulate the quality of health and social care in England by ensuring that all providers meet their requisite standards (CQC 2018). Under their duties provided by section 2 of the Health Act 2009, both are still required to regard the quality of care provided to patients (as well as the principles outlined by the NHS Constitution) in undertaking their organisational regulatory responsibilities.

Each NHS body is required to monitor and put arrangements in place to improve the quality of care provided to service users (Health and Social Care (Community

Health and Standards) Act 2003). The Health Act 2009 further requires all NHS organisations (including Foundation Trusts) to provide information relevant to the quality of their service provision. All providers (whether NHS or private) must be registered with the CQC, and a failure to meet the necessary standards may result in a compliance notice, fine, remedial order or prosecution.

Unlike NHS Trusts, Foundation Trusts have a little more autonomy (particularly concerning financial matters). Derived from the National Health Service Act 2006 (as amended by the Health and Social Care Act 2012), Monitor has the regulatory responsibility for Foundation Trusts.

Northern Ireland

The Regulation and Quality Improvement Authority (RQIA) is the independent body responsible for monitoring and inspecting the availability and quality of health and social care services in Northern Ireland, and encouraging improvements in the quality of those services.

In 2001, the Northern Ireland Executive's Programme for Government included a commitment to raise the quality of public services. *Best Practice, Best Care* (2002) was published by the Department of Health, Social Services and Public Safety (DHSSPS), calling on health and social care organisations to fulfil a statutory duty of quality for the first time. The Health and Personal Social Services (Quality, Improvement and Regulation) (Northern Ireland) Order 2003 created the enabling legal framework for raising the quality of health and social care services in Northern Ireland. The RQIA was established in 2015 as a non-departmental public body of the DHSSPS. Under the Health and Social Care (Reform) Act (Northern Ireland) 2009, the RQIA also began to undertake functions previously carried out by the Mental Health Commission. Unlike in Wales, the RQIA undertakes both health and social care reviews.

The RQIA has various enforcement powers, including non-compliance notices, conditions of registration and prosecutions.

Scotland

Created in 2011 following the Public Services Reform (Scotland) Act 2010, Healthcare Improvement Scotland (HIS) took over from NHS Quality Improvement Scotland to implement the healthcare priorities of the Scottish Government, in particular the Healthcare Quality Strategy of NHS Scotland (Scottish Government 2016). As part of this, HIS:

- develops evidence-based advice, guidance and standards for effective clinical practice
- drives and supports the improvement of healthcare practice
- provides assurance about the quality and safety of healthcare through scrutiny and reporting on performance.

As part of the programme of work, HIS incorporates several organisations:

- The *Healthcare Environment Inspectorate* (HEI) inspects the safety and cleanliness of healthcare services across NHS Scotland and also ensures that the required standards of care are met and areas for improvement are addressed.

- The *Scottish Health Council* improves how NHS Scotland involves patients and the public in decisions about their health.

- The *Scottish Health Technologies Group* provides evidence on the clinical and cost-effectiveness of existing and future technologies to NHS Scotland boards when they consider using health technologies.

- The *Scottish Intercollegiate Guidelines Network* develops and disseminates evidence-based clinical practice guidelines to improve quality of care for patients in Scotland.

- The *Scottish Medicines Consortium* provides advice to NHS boards and Area Drug and Therapeutics Committees (ADTCs) about all newly licensed medicines.

- The *Scottish Patient Safety Programme* launched in 2008 as a five-year programme to reduce hospital standardised mortality ratios to 20%, with the most recently available data indicating a 16.1% reduction in December 2015.

Wales

Healthcare Inspectorate Wales (HIW) inspects NHS services and independent healthcare providers in Wales against a range of standards, policies, guidance and regulations to highlight areas requiring improvement (HIW 2017). Working in a similar way to the CQC and Monitor, HIW reviews services to ensure that they comply with regulations, meet healthcare standards, and that individuals meet their legislative and professional standards and guidance as applicable. Where providers fail to meet the required standard, HIW has various enforcement powers, including non-compliance notices, intensified monitoring, mandatory action plans and criminal prosecutions. It also has the authority to place NHS providers into special measures; however, it can only take this action with the authority of the Welsh Government.

Care and Social Services Inspectorate Wales (CSSIW) regulates social care and social services in Wales, also aiming to provide independent assurance on the quality of services. Where social care providers fail, CSSIW can issue non-compliance notices, suspension of services, suspension of registration and prosecution.

Towards the end of the Fourth Assembly (May 2016), a Welsh Government Green Paper consulted on the need to reconsider the regulation and inspection of healthcare settings in light of a review of Healthcare Inspectorate Wales and the changes proposed by the Regulation and Inspection of Social Care (Wales) Act 2016. This included whether HIW should be merged with CSSIW. However, at the time of writing (February 2019), there is no set plan for this merger in place.

Community Health Councils (CHCs) are statutory bodies that represent the patient and the public in the Welsh NHS. CHCs are intended to develop the links between the public and providers, and have the power to inspect NHS premises and make recommendations for improvement. In 2014, it was recommended that CHCs also be extended to social care; however, this has not yet been pursued by the Welsh Government.

Patient Safety

Recent decades have seen the growing emphasis on a patient safety culture, and a range of initiatives have been developed.

The World Health Organization (WHO) World Alliance for Patient Safety (2005) set out a *Safer Patients* initiative to reduce the incidence of medical error and enhance communication between teams. The initiative focuses on using warning systems to detect signs that the patient may be deteriorating at an early stage.

Hard Truths: The Journey to Putting Patients First was the UK Government's 2013 response to the Mid Staffordshire NHS Foundation Trust Inquiry report (The Stationery Office 2013). This recommends improving patient involvement in care and increasing transparency to enhance patient safety.

In 2015, the NHS launched its Never Events framework. Never Events are serious incidents that are entirely preventable but occur when guidance or safety recommendations are not implemented correctly. The framework outlines how staff providing and commissioning NHS-funded services should identify, investigate and respond to Never Events occurring in clinical practice. Whilst this list may seemingly have little correspondence to paramedic practice, medication events and undetected oesophageal intubation are both listed, and both may affect paramedics in clinical practice as much as any other healthcare professional. Chapter 14 will give a much more thorough overview of the legislation relating to medicines management for paramedics and the correlations this has to improving patient safety.

Learning from Error

In 2005 and 2010, the now-disbanded National Patient Safety Agency (NPSA) published *Medical Error*. These are guidance booklets that provide advice and guidance for junior doctors on preventing and reporting patient safety incidents. In both versions, senior doctors discuss mistakes they have made and how they have learnt from them, and the second (2010) version has key steps outlined for how to report something that does go wrong, including how to handle complaints.

These documents are incredibly important. As well as providing a useful tool for reporting mistakes, they contain stories where mistakes are talked about, the errors made and the lessons learned. Importantly, these examples come from some of the greatest contemporary clinical leaders in medicine, demonstrating that everyone can make mistakes, but it is how they are learned from that results in the development of a safer and more effective healthcare system, both within the NHS and outside of it.

Acknowledging that an error took place requires personal insight, courage and a desire to improve. These are characteristics that are fundamental to the development of individual clinicians within the healthcare setting and that must be supported by the culture overall. The HCPC places great emphasis on the need for honesty amongst its registrants, and a statutory Duty of Candour (a legal obligation and professional responsibility to be honest with patients when things go wrong) applies to all care providers registered with the CQC (regulation 20 of the Health and Social Care Act 2008 (Regulated Activities) Regulations 2014). The intention of this regulation is to ensure that providers are open and transparent with service users and others acting lawfully on their behalf in relation to care and treatment. This regulation also sets out specific requirements for providers to follow when things go wrong with care and treatment, including informing people about the incident, providing support, providing honest information and an apology (Health and Social Care Act 2008).

However, errors can be multi-factorial and may not have a single root cause. Chapter 8 will outline some cases, such as the most recent Bawa-Garba case, where this has occurred. In these instances, root cause analysis allows deficiencies to be revealed at the individual, team and organisational levels. A proactive approach to prevention or reduction of error requires that any weaknesses in the system, whether they be individual or team-based, are addressed in order to avoid error repetition and increase overall patient safety.

Clinical Governance

Clinical governance is 'a system through which NHS organisations are accountable for continuously improving the quality of their services and safeguarding high standards of care by creating an environment in which excellence in clinical care will flourish' (Scally and Donaldson 1998, p. 61). It resonates clearly with the NHS Constitution, with its purpose to maintain patient safety and ensure high-quality healthcare.

Clinical governance is an umbrella term. It covers activities that help sustain and improve high standards of patient care. Healthcare organisations have a duty to maintain the quality and safety of care. Whatever structures, systems and processes an organisation puts in place, it must be able to show evidence that standards are upheld.

It is generally accepted that there are seven elements of clinical governance, which are as follows.

Clinical Audit

Audit is the process by which clinical practice is measured against a set of standards. The standards should be evidence-based and representative of current practice. Findings are then used to implement change and improve care, and the audit is then repeated to measure any improvement attained.

Clinical Effectiveness and Research

Clinical effectiveness is a measure of the extent to which a particular intervention works. The measure on its own is useful, but decisions are enhanced by considering additional factors, such as whether the intervention is appropriate and whether it represents value for money. In the modern health service, clinical practice needs to be refined in the light of emerging evidence of effectiveness, but also has to consider aspects of efficiency and safety from the perspective of individual patients.

Clinical effectiveness should therefore be research-led (or evidence-led). Techniques such as critical appraisal of the literature and the development of clinical guidelines that represent best practice, and implementation strategies to disseminate and implement research, are central to ensuring that patient care is effective and safe.

Education, Training and Continuing Professional Development

It is crucial that education programmes are iterative to sustain the skills of the clinicians they seek to educate. Curriculum content is revised at local (university) levels as well as within the College of Paramedics, which sets the curriculum standards for undergraduate and postgraduate paramedics within the UK. Content should be reflective of the literature, but also complemented with practice – for example, there is currently debate about the place of endotracheal intubation in the paramedic skill set. Practice would indicate that this is a procedure that is rarely performed, except by those acting in critical care roles. Current research is inconclusive regarding the rote ability of paramedics to intubate. Responding to such dilemmas requires curriculums to be updated frequently in order to ensure best practice and patient care.

There is also a duty on the paramedic registrant to manage their professional development. Chapter 2 looks at what this means for paramedics in more detail.

Information Management

Information management in healthcare includes patient records (demographic, socioeconomic and clinical information). The management and use of information within healthcare systems determines the system's effectiveness in detecting health problems, defining priorities, identifying innovative solutions and allocating resources to improve health outcomes. This also crosses over with information governance, which is discussed further in Chapter 5.

Risk Management

Managing risk incorporates two components: identifying risk and managing complaints. Identifying risks within clinical practice is often the most difficult aspect of risk management. Such identification relies on the reporting of adverse events by staff and therefore a culture where reporting is encouraged. Incident reporting should allow significant events to be identified and their level of risk assessed, usually by root cause analysis. These results then enable the production of controls or actions which can be disseminated widely to ensure that risk is reduced in future (Churchill 2008).

However, risk management does not focus on incident reporting alone; it also includes managing complaints. At the centre of efficient quality management is effective complaints handling. Generally, once received, a complaint is dealt with by local resolution within the organisation. Part of this process requires the issues raised by the complaint to be addressed, and the complainant response to include a reflective element or identify learning points with suggestions for future improvement. If the complainant remains dissatisfied, it may be referred to the independent Ombudsman.

Patient and Public Involvement

As within research, involving patients and public in clinical governance requires a multi-faceted approach. Obtaining a wide cross-section of reviews is important in order to produce a balanced viewpoint. Vulnerable groups (such as black and ethnic minorities or adults with learning difficulties) are seldom vocal, and encouragement is often sought to ensure that these groups are able to contribute to the development of the system.

Staffing and Staff Management

It seems obvious that staff who feel valued, supported and informed are more loyal to the environment in which they work. In clinical governance, staffing and staff management focuses on the recruitment, management and development of staff as well as the promotion of good working conditions and effective methods of working. Effective staffing and staff management includes:

- appropriate recruitment of staff
- ensuring that underperformance is identified and addressed
- encouraging staff retention by motivating and developing staff
- providing good working conditions.

Clinical Guidelines

Clinical guidelines are care-based strategies that recommend how healthcare professionals should care for patients in particular circumstances. The development of the guidelines involves the collection and ranking of research and data to ensure that it represents best practice.

The *UK Ambulance Services Clinical Practice Guidelines* provide guidance for NHS paramedics, although the principles are applicable to the work of all those who work in ambulance services. Developed by the Joint Royal Colleges Ambulance Liaison Committee, these guidelines are often fondly (but incorrectly) cited as JRCALC.

A majority of other clinical guidelines have been developed by the National Institute for Health and Care Excellence (NICE), by professional colleges or by specialist societies. Unlike the others, NICE is also tasked to ensure that its guidelines give weight to the best available evidence, as well as the cost-effectiveness of the recommendation advised. There is a growing tendency to measure clinical practice against the established guidelines, something that again features in the discussion of the Bolam test in Chapter 8.

The Law, Ethics and the Paramedic?

It is an incredibly exciting time to be a paramedic. Clinical practice is open to paramedics across military, charity, civilian and business settings. Whether working in the NHS ambulance service, private hospital providers, expedition medicine or retrieval support, the versatility offered by paramedics is finally being recognised across the world. However, this is not without its challenges. Each setting will require a slightly different skill set, a slightly different scope of practice, a slightly different governance structure and a slightly different approach to problems. One constant is the day-to-day issues of the moral and legal contours of the paramedic–patient relationship. Whilst these settings may be different in terms of environment and clinical practice, each is full of its own ethical dilemmas and legal influence, which can sometimes be difficult to navigate. As a profession underpinned by registration, working within education, research and leadership also bring with it the obligations owed in relation to matters of public health. Each pillar of practice brings a similar amount of problems, albeit concerning different ethical and legal principles. Ethics allows the justification of a particular course of action by reference to wider, socially accepted norms or values. An understanding of the law ensures that actions are legally robust and without criticism of negligence. Understanding ethical principles and legal concepts will help clinicians to decide which path is the better option during a difficult decision. Whilst there is more than one 'right' answer, the 'wrong' answer is the path that is not justifiable – both legally and ethically. An understanding of how to navigate such concepts is key to personal and professional development, as well as the continued growth of the paramedic profession as a whole.

How This Book Works

Written by paramedics for paramedics, this book presents an introduction to the law and ethics within paramedic practice. Following the usual academic drill, each chapter author outlines their chosen topic, embraces principles (with a healthy amount of criticism) and draws recommendations for practice and conclusions.

In *Chapter 2*, Ceri Sudron begins by providing a concise history of the paramedic profession, before exploring contemporary practice and the role of the HCPC in the paramedic profession. An introduction to ethical principles underpinning healthcare delivery is presented in *Chapter 3*, in which Georgette Eaton aims to outline different ethical outlooks in order to promote self-reflection in the hope that the reader may develop their own ethical standing. *Chapter 4* by Keiran Bellis presents a more rigid overview of the legal system within the UK. Bellis' aim in this chapter is to introduce the reader to UK law and how it is applicable to practice, with understanding surrounding the differences between the Courts. Keiran continues in *Chapter 5* by explaining the law pertaining to information governance, data protection and confidentiality within paramedic practice. Aidan Baron then lends his voice in *Chapter 6* to applying the legal mechanisms alongside professional and ethical considerations in the professional use of social media. In *Chapter 7*, Vince Clarke outlines the differing types of consent readers may face in practice, discussing the relevant case law and advice. *Chapter 8* covers clinical negligence, in which Edd

Barlett and Georgette Eaton discuss the development of clinical negligence within case law and promote candidacy when faced with medical error. Legislation relating to mental health is explored by Samantha McCabe-Hogan in *Chapter 9*, which aims to give the reader a more solid understanding of the Mental Health Act. Samantha uses real case studies to outline important elements within the evolution of the Act and the resulting treatment considerations. Edd Barlett goes on to explore the Mental Capacity Act 2005 in *Chapter 10*, citing relevant case law to apply it to paramedic practice. The interaction between the Mental Capacity Act and Mental Health Act concludes this chapter and offers a crucial element to understanding; therefore, readers are urged to review Chapters 9 and 10 together. Issues surrounding consent, capacity and negligence for patients under the age of 18 are outlined by Will Broughton and Georgette Eaton in *Chapter 11*.

In *Chapter 12*, dual-registered general practitioner (GP) and paramedic Tom Mallinson focuses on the specific legal and ethical issues pertaining to decision making in palliative and end-of-life care, and the role of the paramedic. The chapter presents the legal and ethical considerations to end-of-life care and the supportive documentation paramedics may encounter. Edd Bartlett kindly presents a note from the writing from his Master's thesis in *Chapter 13*, which considers of uncontrolled organ donation after circulatory death. In *Chapter 14*, an overview of the legal and ethical practice of medicines management within paramedic practice is presented by Andy Collen, as the College of Paramedics Prescribing lead. John Renshaw appeals to aspiring researchers in *Chapter 15*, offering a summary of the reasoning behind medical research ethics and outlining the approval process for health research.

From this brief glimpse ahead, it can be seen that this book presents the essential information about a big issue. Throughout the chapters, case studies will be used to develop further insights into the concepts discussed, and the chapters will include recommendations for practice and recommended further reading for perusal.

> *Points for consideration are presented like this in the main text.*

Learning from the experience of the author team, each with their own interest, specialism or background within these principles, this book presents a guide to applying law and ethics to paramedic practice. No single set of instructions can hope to cover the multitude of experiences, settings, issues and dilemmas a paramedic may face in the diverse range of settings in which they work. As such, in place of a guide, this book will provide an introduction to understanding the essential legal and ethical issues pertinent to paramedic practice.

References

Care Quality Commission (CQC) (2018) *What we do*. Available at: www.cqc.org.uk/what-we-do.

Churchill, D (2008) Putting the principles of good governance into clinical practice. *Obstetrician & Gynaecologist*, 10: 93–98.

Collen, A (2017) *Decision Making in Paramedic Practice*. Bridgwater: Class Professional Publishing.

Department of Health (2015) *NHS Constitution for England*. Available at: www.gov.uk/government/publications/the-nhs-constitution-for-england.

Eaton, G, Mahtani, K and Catterall, M (2018) The evolving role of paramedics: NICE problems to have? *Journal of Health Services Research & Policy*, 23(9): 193–95.

Evans, R, McGovern, R, Birch, J et al. (2013) Which extended paramedic skills are making an impact in emergency care and can be related to the UK paramedic system? A systematic review of the literature. *Emergency Medicine Journal*, 31: 594–603.

Healthcare Inspectorate Wales (HIW) (2017) *What we do*. Available at: http://hiw.org.uk/about/whatwedo/?lang=en.

National Institute for Health and Care Excellence (NICE) (2017) *Consultation*. Chapter 4: Paramedic Remote Support. Available at: www.nice.org.uk/guidance/GID-CGWAVE0734/documents/draft-guideline-4.

O'Meara, P (2014) Community paramedics: a scoping review of their emergence and potential impact. *International Paramedic Practice*, 4: 5–12.

Pearson, B. (2017) The clinical governance of multidisciplinary care. *International Journal of Health Governance*, 22(4): 246–50.

Scally, G and Donaldson, L (1998) Clinical governance and the drive for quality improvement in the new NHS in England. *BMJ*, 317(7150): 61–65.

Scottish Government (2016) *Healthcare Improvement Scotland*. Available at: www.gov.scot/Topics/Health/Quality-Improvement-Performance/HealthCareImprovementScotland.

The Stationery Office (2013) *Report of the Mid Staffordshire NHS Foundation Trust Public Inquiry: Executive Summary*. London: The Stationery Office.

Wankhade, P (2010) *Cultural characteristics in the ambulance service and its relationship with organisational performance: evidence from the UK*. In: Management of Emergency Response Services: Does Culture Matter Track, PAC Conference, 6–8 September 2010, Nottingham Business School, UK.

Williams, B et al. (2013) Next generation paramedics, agents of change, or time for curricula renewal? *Advances in Medical Education and Practice*, 4: 245–50.

World Health Organization (WHO) (2005) *World Alliance for Patient Safety: Safer Patients*. Available at: http://www.who.int/patientsafety/en/brochure_final.pdf.

UK Legislation

Health and Social Care Act 2008

Chapter 2

A Concise History of the Paramedic Profession

Ceri Sudron

If we can understand what we do, develop a robust knowledge base, be true to ourselves and have a sense of the future, we can truly become a profession in our own right.

(O'Meara 2009, p. 57)

Introduction

Prior to the 1970s, ambulance services in the UK were predominantly voluntary services provided by individual hospitals. Scotland has the earliest recorded recognised service as early as 1775, with Staffordshire General being one of the first to be recognised in England in the 1800s and Liverpool boasting a horse-drawn service serving the Northern Hospital in 1884 (Liverpool Medical Institution 2017). It wasn't until the National Health Service Act 1946 that local authorities across the UK were expected to provide dedicated Local Authority Ambulance Services where necessary, for the conveyance of persons suffering illness or mental defectiveness or expectant or nursing mothers (National Health Service Act 1946).

What's in a Name?

The earliest mention of the word 'paramedic' is from 1911 (Aronson 2017) with the prefix 'para' meaning *related to* or *working alongside*. Prior to the 1990s, the word 'paramedical' was at first used to denote those working alongside the medic (the physician), becoming a noun, then a name. Thus, the paramedic emerged. The original term 'paramedic' could be used for anyone who was not a doctor but was involved in the medical care and included social workers and members of the clergy. By 1990, it became the term used for non-doctors engaged in pre-hospital and emergency care.

The humble beginnings of the paramedic profession are argued to have begun with the Miller Report of 1964, in which recommendations for ambulance services to treat rather than just transport patients were outlined. The first 'extended training schemes' began in Brighton in 1971 under the stewardship of cardiologist Dr (now Professor) Douglas Chamberlain (College of Paramedics 2017a). Dr Peter Baskett, a consultant anaesthetist, followed with a similar scheme in Bristol the following year, and other pilot schemes spread across the UK during the early 1970s (College of Paramedics 2017a). The first recognised performance standards came a decade later in 1974, when responsibility for the ambulance service moved from the local authority to NHS control (Pollock 2012).

Under the control of the NHS, ambulance services continued to develop, with ambulance drivers requiring a first aid certificate in order to provide initial treatment prior to transport to definitive care. In 1981, a National Health Service Training Authority (NHSTA) was formed to provide the extended care ambulance staff course, which in 1985 was endorsed by the Department of Health to become the nationally recognised course for locally trained paramedics (College of Paramedics 2017b). The NHSTA courses eventually became the Institute of Health and Care Development (IHCD), awarding ambulance care assistant, ambulance technician and ambulance paramedic vocational qualifications until it was taken over by Edexcel in 1998 and Pearson in 2004. Courses continued to be delivered in this guise until they were discontinued in 2006.

These initial developments in the education and training of staff working in the ambulance service gradually led to the role of the paramedic as it is known today. Whilst vocational training began in 1985, paramedic education started within higher education in 1996, with the first UK undergraduate paramedic degree starting at the University of Hertfordshire. From 1 September 2021, new student paramedics will only be able to start degree-level programmes (HCPC 2018a).

Defining a Profession

A profession historically dates back to medieval ages and was usually reserved for lawyers, the clergy and doctors (First et al. 2012), yet today many more occupations meet the criteria of a profession by virtue of requiring the individual to exhibit autonomy, self-direction, accountability and education (Bossers et al. 1999). A profession is now regarded as an occupation that embodies an element of trust and the need for honesty and confidentiality, particularly in relation to patient information (Burford et al. 2011; Evetts 2013).

Developing into a profession, paramedics became the twelfth Allied Health Profession with compulsory professional registration with the Council for Professions Supplementary to Medicine in 2000, which subsequently evolved into the Health Professions Council in 2003 (and has since been renamed as the HCPC in 2012). However, registration was more than just a legally recognised title, its primary aim being to protect service users, their families, carers and other practitioners from unprofessional practice (Woollard 2009).

Registration with the HCPC also guaranteed a standardised level of competence with adherence to Standards of Practice uniting the profession across the many different settings in which paramedics may be employed. With HCPC registration and adherence to the *Standards of Proficiency* (HCPC 2014) and the *Standards of Conduct, Performance and Ethics* (HCPC 2016a) comes accountability, self-regulation and responsibility for both individual and profession-wide conduct.

With inclusion on the HCPC register, and the formation of the Joint Royal Colleges Ambulance Liaison Committee (JRCALC), paramedicine has become a profession in its own right with nationally accepted guidelines, more autonomy and self-direction (Evetts 2013). Modern paramedic practice lays greater emphasis on decision making, accountability and best practice for individual patients rather than on strict adherence to local protocols. This move to a profession also necessitated the formation of a professional body and the British Paramedic Association was founded in 2001, becoming the College of Paramedics in 2009. Today, a registered charity, it remains the voice of the developing paramedic profession.

Law, Ethics and the Paramedic

All professions demand adherence to ethics and law, this itself necessitating extended education in order to practise with knowledge, skill and competence that is maintained by the individual. From the humble beginnings of horse-drawn volunteers to convey sick people to hospital, to the profession of autonomous clinicians that we see now, paramedics are marked out by their generalist knowledge and the autonomy of their actions, which demands accountability and ethical considerations within an evidence- and values-based framework.

Contemporary Practice

Values-based

The HCPC commissioned a report in 2012 to explore professionalism across three registered professions, one of which was paramedicine. This report determined that professionalism in terms of definition is context-dependent and that there is subjectivity due to the individual practitioner, the patient and the setting. Professionalism is dictated by internalised values, attitudes and ethical behaviour that are personal to the practitioner, therefore being innate rather than taught (HCPC 2012b).

Values in healthcare are more often based on medical ethics such as beneficence and non-malevolence (Beauchamp and Childress 2013); however, this also encompasses needs, preferences, wishes, personal expression, evaluation and judgements (Fulford 2011). Values are highly personal – we all have them, professions have them and organisations have them – but sometimes personal values do not match what the profession or the organisation claims. Therefore, values-based practice operates as a twin framework to evidence-based practice to ensure that professional values encompass both who and what we profess to be (Fulford 2011).

Within the paramedic context, behaviours that *may* constitute professionalism are encompassed in arguably nebulous terms such as altruism, advocacy, excellence and humanism. Values that align with these behaviours are not necessarily exhibited by all paramedics, given that values are highly subjective, intensely personal and often conflict (Eaton 2018). Notions such as confidentiality, best interest and capacity are clear practice terms; however, the enactment of them at the patient's side can be complex, which is likely due to the values of the patient and the clinician. There can be conflict with the practitioner's internal values and their need to disclose information or work in a particular manner to achieve gold standard care (Fulford 2011).

Professionalism should begin with the individual and extend to practice that reflects both occupational and organisational values (Stern et al. 2005). Perhaps more importantly, there needs to be a realisation of the diversity and the complexity of terms such as values, attitudes and behaviours. There is an acknowledgement within the published literature that paramedics have not yet fully realised a status of professionalism, due in part to such things as organisational culture that prohibit this enactment of professional values, ethics and behaviours (O'Meara 2009; McCann et al. 2013). Values-based practice looks to outline the understanding of values as a theoretical basis before then empowering the realisation of values within the clinical setting (Fulford 2011).

Professionalism

Professionalism as a concept is complex and often subjective, and is couched in altruistic terms that mean little to the individual practitioner. The professionalisation of the role of the paramedic is best summarised by First et al. (2012, p. 378), who suggest a process whereby practitioners with a level of education, skills and behaviour 'close the market' so that only similarly qualified practitioners can then assume both the title and the role. The six domains of professionalism given in Table 2.1 are altruistic terms that, when unpicked, can be seen to be echoed throughout the literature of the HCPC and by paramedics themselves. In the *Consensus towards Understanding and Sustaining Professionalism in Paramedic Practice Project* (CUSPPP), both qualified paramedics and paramedic students agreed that professional behaviour needed to encompass responsibility and accountability. These individual qualities of social responsibility, respect and ethical practice may be innate, but can arguably be better enhanced through education. However, the enactment of professionalism based on these qualities is practice-dependent and is influenced by individual values and beliefs (Gallagher et al. 2016; Eaton 2018). In short, professionalism is grown and not made (Burford et al. 2014).

When considering the professionalisation of the paramedic role, core values and behaviours that are considered to constitute professionalism have been previously

Table 2.1   Six Domains of Professionalism (Hilton and Slotnick 2005)

Six domains of professionalism
Responsibility and accountability
Reflection/self-awareness
Social responsibility
Respect for patients
Teamwork
Ethical practice

outlined (O'Meara 2009; McCann et al. 2013; The Stationery Office 2013), aligning with the *Standards of Proficiency* (HCPC 2014) and the *Standards of Conduct, Performance and Ethics* (HCPC 2016a) outlined by the HCPC. Professional behaviour encompasses everything from personal presentation and benevolence through to individuals advancing the profession. This all translates into practice as paramedics being directed to put the patient's best interests foremost in all their decisions, their performance, their behaviour, their attitude, their communication and their endeavour to provide the patient with the best-quality experience. However, it is not just registered paramedics who fall within professional boundaries. These principles also apply to the professionalisation of the paramedic workforce, thus encompassing all employees of all grades from student to entry level, through to chief executives (Wagner et al. 2007).

Professionalism is a concept that, whilst it starts with regulation and registration, pertains to the quality of care given, the level of competence held by the clinician and ultimately the passion and pride in the delivery of quality care (Scottish Government 2012). Both professionalism and values-based practice interlink, with the definition of fitness to practise being as follows: 'having the skills, knowledge and character to practise safely and effectively' (HCPC 2016a, p. 6). Inherent individual values and beliefs may predispose an individual towards professional behaviour; however, the ability to understand one's own values and to apply them within a values-based practice framework would suggest that this is more a determinant of individual rather than organisational competency.

Actions-Based

The catalogue of serious adverse events at the Mid Staffordshire Hospital suggested that there must be a focus upon training for professionalism, an assurance of the possession of appropriate attitudes and behaviours that aligns with both the code and expression of meritorious practice (First et al. 2012; The Stationery Office 2013). Professionalism encompasses individual self-awareness, values and key attributes that put the professional second to the needs of the patient, and the quality of the care they are giving. Therefore, the expectation is for a professional to embody the drive to excel, to continually develop their skills, knowledge and attitudes to ensure professionalism of care at all times (The Stationery Office 2013). Known colloquially as the Francis Report (2013), this report recognised that the professional values of individual practitioners had become compromised by a culture of collusion, silence and acceptance of poor practice. Thus, self-awareness, honesty and values-based practice are key to ensuring an occupational culture of professionalism, and therefore become action-based.

Noordegraaf (2011) outlines three main areas that need to be examined in order to promote a culture of awareness, honesty and professionalism:

- *Cognitive areas*
  These include education, knowledge, skills, confidence and evidence-based healthcare.

- *Normative mechanisms*
  These include entry criteria to education and professional registration, certification of continuing professional development, codes of conduct and disciplinary procedures.

- *Symbolic mechanisms*
  These are set out as cultural rites of passage, interpersonal communication, story-telling, personal codes of ethics, service ideals and missions.

As posited by Gallagher et al. (2016) as part of the CUSPPP, students and paramedics alike continued to highlight the importance of regulation as a normative mechanism and a key component of professionalism. This part of the CUSPPP suggested that professionalism for paramedics – in the eyes of clinicians – was about following the standards of the HCPC and that 'you can't go far wrong because they are the people that tell you what a paramedic essentially is, and if you don't follow their rules you can't call yourself a paramedic' (Gallagher et al. 2016, p. 4). Although simplistic, this statement sums up the necessity of regulation in determining that individuals do meet levels of competence, decision making, attitudes and behaviours.

Whilst the cognitive and normative areas may be set out within a curriculum from the professional body, or standards for registration, the symbolic area often has little uniformity, but offers great importance. The stories that paramedics tell, the behaviour they applaud as being a good clinician and the rites of passage are key to full acceptance as a clinician within the profession, as well as the professionalisation of all grades of staff. This implies a need to look more closely at the organisational culture in which our professional practice sits: do we tell stories and applaud behaviour that matches up to the professionalism we seek?

Mason et al. (2014) have published the Professionalism Charter which allows students within the allied health disciplines (such as paramedicine) to evidence their growth within personal and the interpersonal areas – two elements set within symbolic mechanisms. The Charter (see Table 2.2) defines the construct of professionalism in a way that allows students to plot their strengths and weaknesses within a framework, demonstrating achievement of standards of professional behaviour both in and out of practice.

Table 2.2   Allied Health Professions professionalism charter

Responsibility	Description
Honesty and integrity	The ability to be fair, truthful to keeping one's word and straightforward
Empathy and compassion	The ability to be sensitive and respond to the feelings and behaviours of others
Altruism and respect for others	The ability to demonstrate a commitment to patients, the profession and society through ethical practice

Table 2.2 Allied Health Professions professionalism charter (*continued*)

Responsibility	Description
Trustworthiness and dependability	The capacity to demonstrate reliability and honour commitments
Initiative	The capacity to create and initiate ideas
Judgement	The ability to make wise decisions
Confidentiality	Appropriate safeguarding of the disclosure of patient information
Maintain appropriate relationships with service users	The commitment to avoid inappropriate relationships with patients or their carers
Professional presentation	The ability to present oneself in a manner acceptable to clients, peers and colleagues
Co-operation	The ability to work effectively with others, honouring commitments and being loyal to decisions made
Organisation	The ability to systematically manage tasks, manage oneself and manage others
Responsibility	The commitment to having a responsibility to society, to the profession and to oneself
Commitment to improve	The ability and will to strive for excellence
Competence	Commitment to competence in technical knowledge and skills, ethical and legal obligations and communication skills
Effective verbal communication	The ability to share information with clarity and quality of content
Effective written communication	The ability to communicate information clearly and concisely in written form
Self-awareness	The ability to be insightful, particularly about the state of one's knowledge, skills and behaviours
Supervision	The ability to modify performance in response to meaningful feedback
Reflective practice	The ability to reflect on one's own behaviour and the underlying dynamics and to develop learning as a result
Clinical reasoning	The ability to analyse, synthesise and interpret information

The creation of a professional organisational culture is important in terms of raising the expectations and professionalism of a paramedic, regardless of the employment setting. In moving the profession forward, the behaviour, values and beliefs preventing unprofessional behaviour and the culture of the past must be challenged.

The Francis Report highlighted concerns that the NHS can be an organisation of collusion, outlining silence in the face of poor practice that resulted in patient harm (The Stationery Office 2013). An HCPC report (2016b) concluded that there were still elements of acceptance of poor practice within the ambulance service, compounded by a culture of not speaking out due to fear that other practitioners would then ostracise the complainant. A more recent report has compiled a set of recommendations to overcome a culture of bullying and sexual harassment within the ambulance services in England (NHS Employers 2018). It is evident that such a culture highlights a gross misunderstanding of what it actually means to be professional. Professionalism at all levels and in all roles involves the raising of concern, not only for the patient, but also for colleagues. In doing so, self-awareness, responsibility and individual accountability are maintained. Whilst it is unlikely that any paramedic would intentionally set out to harm patients and colleagues, professionalism encourages a culture of awareness and openness – of learning from errors to enhance clinicians' abilities rather than punishment for making mistakes.

> **Tips for Practice**
> *Consider how you would demonstrate your professional behaviours.*

Whilst registration may be synonymous with professionalism, failure to adhere to the standards expected of registration may result in disciplinary proceedings. The HCPC process of investigation of complaints is not intended to be inherently punitive and is explored in detail below.

HCPC Professional Regulation and Accountability

Exploration of the HCPC Tribunal archives and Fitness to Practice Annual reports indicates that paramedics as a profession have the second highest number of concerns raised (HCPC 2018b), with the majority of these concerns coming through self-referral. More importantly, they also have one of the highest rates of closed concerns that do not progress, as the concern does not meet the criteria or threshold for the standard of acceptance for fitness to practise hearing (HCPC 2016b).

Despite this, within many practice environments, the HCPC may be discussed in terms usually reserved for a headmaster, a regimental sergeant major or a similar authority figure who demands absolute adherence to a code of behaviour. In fact, the ethos of the HCPC is not one of punishment, but of regulation and registration to assure the public of a level of competence from individual clinicians (HCPC 2012a). The HCPC, alongside individual employers, uses policy, procedure, standards and guidelines to outline the expectations of the registrant within any working environment. However, whilst these systems are designed to reduce error of judgements, they are not infallible and it should be remembered that paramedics, particularly those who work in pre-hospital emergency settings, are exposed to a level of risk not experienced in other areas of healthcare (Shaban et al. 2004).

The *Standards of Proficiency* (HCPC 2014) and the *Standards of Conduct, Performance and Ethics* (HCPC 2016a) are designed as a framework of expectations of character, skill and personal attributes to ensure consistency in terms of public expectations for paramedic practice. The expectations are not onerous and apply to all paramedics, regardless of the employment setting.

All registrants (and arguably anyone who contacts patients) should be mindful of how they behave, how they communicate and the need to be honest when things go wrong. Human judgement and decision making is never infallible (Collen 2017); it is always subjective, can be flawed and always carries with it an inherent risk of error that may well affect the patient (Shaban et al. 2004). Registered paramedics should not fear being held accountable to the standards expected of the profession, and these expectations are mirrored across other health professions, including doctors, nurses, physiotherapists and social workers.

The Health and Care Professions Tribunal Service

If a concern is passed to the HCPC, an initial investigation is undertaken. If the Standard of Acceptance is met, the case will be allocated to a case manager in the HCPC's investigations team. The team will gather evidence to make a full assessment of the allegation. The case manager will manage the case through to the Investigating Committee Panel (ICP). The ICP will consider the case and determine whether the case should be closed at that stage, or whether there is a case to answer and it should be referred for a hearing. If there is a case to answer, it is passed to the fitness to practise adjudication service of the Health and Care Professions Council, the Health and Care Professions Tribunal Service (HCPTS). Hearings are conducted and managed by independent panels which are set away from the HCPC. Both the HCPC investigative process and the HCPTS operate within Part V of the *Health and Social Work Professions Order 2001*, and as such are responsible for the safety and assurance of patient care. Therefore, being struck from the register is a first action reserved for only the most heinous mistake, criminal or illegal proceedings, or failure to disclose significant issues of suitability or inability to practise.

Mess room folklore would suggest that the HCPC is keen to strike people from the register, and anecdotal evidence supports this idea of paramedics operating from a position of 'it is my ticket' and the fear of losing it. However, the HCPC in its *Standards* (HCPC 2014, 2016a) and within its own report on professionalism (HCPC 2012b) suggests that its interest is not necessarily focused on the mistake, but on what a professional does with the mistake. The HCPC (2014, 2016a) promotes a culture of accountability and honesty around a practitioner's own behaviour, actions and decisions. If previous and upcoming cases before the HCPTS are reviewed, many allegations concern the decision making regarding the patient's care and the learning associated with the mistake made.

The case of *HCPC v Fisher* (2017) highlights the need for individual self-awareness and accountability for skill. The registrant was suspended as the paramedic did not undertake an adequate assessment or adequately complete documentation for Patient A, or complete documentation for Child A and failed to arrange appropriate referral or safeguarding. The paramedic's length of service was taken into account, but a lack of responsibility for skills erosion and poor decision making was acknowledged. The decision to not complete adequate paperwork was a key finding, being a core expectation of a registered professional's practice. The findings of this case was that the paramedic lacked insight into the seriousness of his failings and two vulnerable service users had been put at risk. In summarising the case, the panel stated that in deciding upon the sanction of suspension, they were mindful of not being seen to punish, but to protect the public.

This case is a good example of how these processes focus on protecting patients rather than punishing clinicians. The process should allow the individual professional to show accountability, responsibility and the values of honesty, candidness and insight or self-awareness.

A different case outlines a different outcome for a failure to complete adequate documentation. In *HCPC v Edwards* (2015), the paramedic received a caution for a drug error and dishonest conduct. These serious events were found to be mitigated by the following points:

- The exceptionally high degree of insight achieved by the Registrant.

- The genuine remorse and contrition shown by the Registrant throughout the course of this hearing has also been exceptional.

- His openness and unconditional acceptance of responsibility for his actions.

- The positive testimonials submitted by persons of standing.

- His voluntary actions in participating in a paramedic training course allowing others to learn from his mistakes.

The findings, even within a serious case of falsely documenting administered drugs and attempted concealment, acknowledged the registrant's attempts to rectify mistakes, take responsibility and show insight. Due to the registrant's insight, remedial behaviour and reflection, the panel were satisfied that the reoccurrence of such behaviour was unlikely, even given the seriousness of the original referral. They concluded that a Conditions of Practice Order or even a Suspension Order would be disproportionate given the paramedic's behaviour in attempting to rectify mistakes and take responsibility, and that a caution was therefore appropriate.

In *HCPC v Garnham* (2018), the registrant failed to ensure that a disconnected 999 call was followed up correctly after contact with the caller was lost. The caller was the patient and this error of judgement and process resulted in their death. The panel decided to afford an opportunity for the registrant to remedy his mistake and be able to demonstrate insight and responsibility, so a Suspension Order was given for 12 months. At the review hearing, it was recorded that the registrant now gave evidence that was honest, detailed and showed his acceptance of accountability and responsibility for his actions. The notes from the case specifically attest to the registrant admitting his defensiveness and previous misconduct in not accepting that he was at fault. It was therefore noted that the registrant now evidenced insight into his own behaviour, showed self-awareness and acceptance of responsibility, and accountability for his actions. In being allowed the time to remedy his mistakes, the registrant was afforded the opportunity to show that there was little risk of repetition and therefore the HCPTS decided on a course of no further action.

In the eyes of the HCPC, responsibility and accountability are fundamental elements of registration. Therefore, if a mistake is made, professional development to overcome the knowledge gap, lack of competence or episodes of poor decision making that resulted in a mistake is crucial in order to retain registration.

Professional Regulation and Accountability in the Ambulance Service: Is it Only for Paramedics?

The HCPC is not a registration body to be feared and it is worth remembering that registration as a paramedic is about protection: of patients, of practitioners and of the title of paramedic. Without this adherence to a minimum standard, the foundation of a recognised profession would not be a reality.

Examination of the relevant case law from the ambulance service in particular demonstrates that there is an expectation for all clinicians to adhere to minimum standards, professional behaviour and common-sense approaches.

Inadequate assessment alongside a failure to take responsibility to exercise a duty of care was seen as a key element in *Choudhury v South Central Ambulance Service NHS Trust and Portsmouth Hospitals NHS Trust* (2015). In this case, two paramedics were dispatched to Mr Choudhury and both misdiagnosed and therefore incorrectly treated his condition. The initial symptoms were of head pains, for which the first paramedic did not record a diagnosis. The second paramedic diagnosed hyperventilation, although the patient was now also vomiting, and this was recorded as food poisoning. There were also serious failings once the patient arrived at hospital nearly 12 hours after the initial onset of symptoms. The treatment of the patient was so significantly delayed by the failings of both the paramedics and the hospital that the basilar artery occlusion the patient was suffering from resulted in both brainstem and cerebellar infarction and locked-in syndrome.

The case of *King v Sussex Ambulance NHS Trust* (2002) highlights the complex relationship between the employer's duty of care to both the employee and the patient. When a non-registered clinician was injured, the judgement acknowledged that whilst the ambulance service must adhere to procedure and standards to enable safe practice, the onus is also on the decision making of the practitioner to complete risk assessments and make sound decisions for themselves.

In the case of *London Ambulance Service NHS Trust v S Small* (2009), the registrant was dismissed for gross misconduct in relation of his handling of an elderly patient. Whilst the claimant exercised his right of appeal, the decision to dismiss was upheld. An employment tribunal subsequently concluded that the dismissal was procedurally unfair, despite the clinical failings of the registrant. After subsequently going through an Employment Appeal Tribunal (UKEAT/0395/07), this case went to the Court of Appeal. The Court of Appeal then advised that whilst its place is not to tell tribunals how to write their judgements, as a general rule it might be better practice in unfair dismissal cases for employment tribunals to keep their findings for liability purposes separate from any findings on disputed issues that are only relevant to other matters, such as clinical competency in this case.

Pause for Thought

Should registration be opened up to include other roles within emergency and unscheduled care?

Should all ambulance staff and first responders be adhering to a recognised minimum standard of care?

Another contested employment tribunal involved an Emergency Medical Technician (EMT) who was not investigated by the HCPC as they were not a registered clinician. In *East of England Ambulance Service NHS Trust v Sanders* (2016), the employment tribunal was contested as the EMT was dismissed following the Trust's internal investigation. In the employment appeal tribunal, the judge highlighted that all clinicians were responsible for their patient care and that the EMT's excuse of being turned down for paramedic training and lack of extended education 'did not excuse her poor patient care'. This case highlights why registration for non-paramedic roles, particularly within the ambulance service, would be of value. The claimant in this case was tasked with taking a patient to hospital after they had been seen by a GP with a suspected hip fracture. In brief, there were a catalogue of attitudinal problems and the crew did not transfer the patient to hospital, where he was later discovered to have suffered a fractured hip. The judge in this case highlighted that all healthcare professionals operate under an assumption of skill, knowledge and behaviour encompassed within the concept of a duty of care. Other healthcare professionals, patients and their relatives, and the public at large have an assumption or expectation of the care that should be delivered by generic ambulance staff. This concept of a benchmark of behaviour, of a need for quality regardless of role within a service is a key element of registration, and therefore would provide a clear and distinguishable framework for all healthcare clinicians.

Whilst training and education may be relevant to professionalism, these cases highlight the importance of individual responsibility for the failure to behave in accordance with organisational expectations. All clinical staff are required to enact a degree of professionalism in order to promote quality patient care. Defining quality expectations from the patient, members of the public and other clinical professionals is what the HCPC was set up to achieve, and to meet expectations is the mark of professionalism. Thus, non-paramedic clinicians such as medical technicians, emergency care assistants, students, apprentices and voluntary community first responders should be held accountable to a base level of professional competence, behaviour and quality of care. The case law explored above demonstrates that the courts see a clear duty of care, and a certain level of competence and behaviour, is expected from all those working in the ambulance service and not just registered paramedics. This behaviour, skill and duty of care commensurate with that of a professional should be demanded of non-registered staff too. These elements of competence, duty of care, decision making, behaviour and attitudes are what all those who work in healthcare delivery are judged against, and so is it time that we enhance the value of paramedic registration and explore levels of registration for the different grades of staff within the ambulance service? Registration of all grades of ambulance staff, rather than just paramedics, would potentially assure the quality of care, a level of competence and the enactment of professional behaviour at all levels of the organisation. Registration with the HCPC should be seen as an embodiment of professionalism, the ability to show professional competence, professional growth and an overall commitment to continually raising the quality of care for the patient.

Summary

The paramedic profession should be applauded for its march towards professionalism. Professionalism is a complex construct that is not simply dictated by organisational culture or professional standards, but is often more thoroughly aligned with the internalised values and attitudes of the individual practitioner. These internalised values and ethics should be enhanced through values-based practice and actively encouraged through a professional culture.

It is imperative that individual paramedics understand the importance of professionalism across the whole context of practice. Professionalism extends from the individual context to the interpersonal context and the organisational culture. However, for individual paramedics, the concept of professionalism is complex and varied, and the societal or organisational expression of professionalism is very much dictated by the organisational culture (Burford et al. 2014). Perhaps we also need to consider the professionalisation of all staff under this umbrella who contribute to patient care. Registration for other members of frontline staff working within the ambulance service may enable professionalism to grow in all contexts of practice. Professionalism demands that quality patient care be placed at the forefront of practice, and that individual practitioners show self-awareness, behaviours and attitudes that align with this. The creation of a professional identity or organisational culture must raise the expectations and professional behaviour of all ambulance roles; the culture of the past and unprofessional behaviour must be challenged so that all healthcare practitioners are mindful of their behaviour and communication, and are honest in their practice.

In contrast to the anecdotal fear of *losing my ticket*, the HCPC supports and encourages responsibility, accountability, personal reflection and the idea that mistakes may be made, but it is the response and the actions following that mistake that determine the HCPC's involvement. Where registrants take responsibility and make themselves accountable, then the HCPC judgement is proportionate and supportive rather than punitive. Paramedics should not fear being held accountable for behaviour, attitudes and judgements, since human decision making is subjective, dictated by context and often flawed (Collen 2017). There is an inherent risk of error within patient care and therefore frameworks, guidelines and standards should guide all clinicians towards making the appropriate judgements. With this in mind, individual paramedics should not fear registration, but should embrace it as a mark of quality, competence and qualification.

Recommended Reading

Fulford, KWM (2011) The value of evidence and evidence of values: bringing together values-based and evidence-based practice in policy and service development in mental health. *Journal of Evaluation in Clinical Practice*, 17: 378–81.

Mason, R et al. (2014) Knowing about and performing professionalism: developing professionalism in interprofessional healthcare education. *International Journal of Practice-Based Learning in Health and Social Care*, **2**(1): 96–107.

McCann, L et al. (2013) Still blue-collar after all these years? An ethnography of the professionalization of emergency ambulance work. *Journal of Management Studies*, 50(5): 749–76.

References

Aronson, J (2017) When I use a word … paramedics. *BMJ Blogs*, 1 December. Available at: https://blogs.bmj.com/bmj/2017/12/01/jeffrey-aronson-when-i-use-a-word-paramedics.

Beauchamp, T and Childress, J (2013) *Principles of Biomedical Ethics*, 7th ed. Oxford: Oxford University Press.

Bossers, A et al. (1999) Defining and developing professionalism. *Canadian Journal of Occupational Therapy*, 66: 116-121.

Burford, B et al. (2011) *Professionalism and conscientiousness in healthcare professionals*. Progress report for Study 2 – Development of quantitative approaches to professionalism. Medical Education Research Group, School of Medicine and Health, Durham University. Available at: https://www.hcpc-uk.org/globalassets/resources/reports/measuring-professionalism-as-a-multi-dimensional-construct---professionalism-and-conscientiousness-in-healthcare-professionals---study-2.pdf.

Burford, B et al. (2014) Professionalism education should reflect reality: findings from three health professions. *Medical Education in Review*, 48(4): 361–74.

College of Paramedics (2017a) *The journey of the College*. Available at: http://www.collegeof paramedics.co.uk/about_us/the-journey-of-the-college.

College of Paramedics (2017b) *Paramedic Curriculum Guidance*, 4th ed. Bridgwater: College of Paramedics.

Collen, A (2017) *Decision Making in Paramedic Practice*. Bridgwater: Class Professional Publishing.

Department of Health (2005) *Taking Healthcare to the Patient: Transforming NHS Ambulance Services*. London: Department of Health.

Eaton, G (2018) How does the practicum for paramedic students impact on the development of their professional values? (Master's thesis). Available at: www.researchgate.net/publication/330311654_How_Does_the_Practicum_for_Paramedic_Students_Impact_on_The_Development_of_Their_Professional_Values.

Evetts, J (2013) Professionalism: value and ideology. *Current Sociology*. Available at: http://csi.sagepub.com/content/early/2013/03/22/0011392113479316.1.

First, S, Tomlins, L and Swinburn, A (2012) From trade to profession: the professionalisation of the paramedic workforce. *Journal of Paramedic Practice*, 4(7): 378–81.

Fulford, KWM (2011) The value of evidence and evidence of values: bringing together values-based and evidence-based practice in policy and service development in mental health. *Journal of Evaluation in Clinical Practice*, 17: 378–81.

Gallagher, A et al. (2016) Professionalism in paramedic practice: the views of paramedics and paramedic students. *British Paramedic Journal*, 1(2): 1–8.

Health and Care Professions Council (HCPC) (2012a) *Why Your HCPC Registration Matters*. London: HCPC.

Health and Care Professions Council (HCPC) (2012b) *Professionalism in Healthcare Professionals. Research Report*. London: HCPC.

Health and Care Professions Council (HCPC) (2014) *Standards of Proficiency – Paramedics*. London: HCPC.

Health and Care Professions Council (HCPC) (2016a) *Standards of Conduct, Performance and Ethics*. London: HCPC.

Health and Care Professions Council (HCPC) (2016b) *Fitness to Practise Annual Report 2016*. London: HCPC.

Health and Care Professions Council (HCPC) (2018a) *HCPC decision on threshold level of qualification for paramedics*. Available at: www.hcpc-uk.org/news-and-events/news/2018/hcpc-decision-on-threshold-level-of-qualification-for-paramedics.

Health and Care Professions Council (HCPC) (2018b) *Fitness to Practice Annual Report 2018*. Available at: www.hcpc-uk.org/resources/reports/2018/fitness-to-practise-annual-report-2018.

Hilton, S. and Slotnick, H (2005) Proto-professionalism: how professionalisation occurs across the continuum of medical education. *Medical Education 39: 58–65*.

Liverpool Medical Institution (2017) *Timeline of ambulance development*. Available at: www.evolve360.co.uk/lmi/Default.aspx.

Mason, R et al. (2014) Knowing about and performing professionalism: developing professionalism in interprofessional healthcare education. *International Journal of Practice-Based Learning in Health and Social Care*, 2(1): 96–107.

McCann, L et al. (2013) Still blue-collar after all these years? An ethnography of the professionalization of emergency ambulance work. *Journal of Management Studies*, 50(5): 749–76.

NHS Employers (2018) *Tackling bullying in ambulance trusts: a guide for action*. Available at: www.nhsemployers.org/your-workforce/plan/ambulance-workforce/tackling-bullying.

Noordegraaf, M (2011) Remaking professionals? How associations and professional education connect professionalism and organisations. *Current Sociology*, 59: 465–88.

O'Meara, P (2009) Paramedics marching towards professionalism. *Australasian Journal of Paramedicine*, 7(1). Available at: https://ajp.paramedics.org/index.php/ajp/article/view/153/165.

Pollock, A (2012) Ambulance services in London and Great Britain from 1860 until today: a glimpse of history gleaned mainly from the pages of contemporary journals. *Emergency Medicine Journal*, 30(3): 218–22.

Scottish Government (2012) *Professionalism in Nursing, Midwifery and the Allied Health Professions in Scotland: A Report to the Coordinating Council for the NNMAHP Contribution to the Healthcare Quality Strategy for NHS Scotland.* Available at: www.gov.scot/resource/0039/00396525.pdf.

Shaban, R et al. (2004) Uncertainty, error and risk in human clinical judgment: introductory theoretical frameworks in paramedic practice. *Journal of Emergency Primary Health Care,* 2(1) DOI: 10.33151/ajp.2.1.263.

Stern, DT, Frohna, AZ and Gruppen, LD (2005) The prediction of professional behaviour. *Medical Education,* 39: 75–82.

The Stationery Office (2013) *Report of the Mid Staffordshire NHS Foundation Trust Public Inquiry: Executive Summary.* London: The Stationery Office.

Wagner, P et al. (2007) Defining medical professionalism: a qualitative study. *Medical Education,* 41: 288–94.

Woollard M (2009) Professionalism in UK paramedic practice. *Journal of Emergency Primary Health Care,* 7(4): Article 990390.

UK Cases

Choudhury v South Central Ambulance Service NHS Trust and Portsmouth Hospitals NHS Trust [2015] EWHC 1311, QB

East of England Ambulance Service NHS Trust v Sanders [2016] UKEAT 0319_15_1102

King v Sussex Ambulance NHS Trust [2002] EWCA Civ 953

London Ambulance Service NHS Trust v S Small [2009] EWCA Civ 220

HCPC Cases

HCPC v Edwards (2015)

HCPC v Fisher (2017)

HCPC v Garnham (2018)

Chapter 3

An Introduction to Ethics

Georgette Eaton

Ethical discourse is concerned with the search for justification for our actions

(Laurie, Harmon and Porter 2016: 5)

Introduction

Ethics (also known as moral philosophy) is concerned with how people *ought* to act and how people *conduct* themselves towards achieving a *good life* – a life that is worth living. Here is the first hurdle in theorising about ethics – not everyone will agree on the principles that govern good conduct or a good life, and there are many different views on what makes a life 'good'. It should not be thought that ethics is necessarily about discovering what is 'right' or 'good', but instead as a vehicle to explore the nature of morality.

Ethics differ from morals, in that ethics denotes the theory of something that is right, whereas morals indicate their practice. Ethics also differ from values, where actions are treated as abstract ideas. Both morals and values deal with the right conduct and living a good life, but what makes an action morally driven or value-driven depends on the whole of a person's ideals and behaviours – their *weltanschauung* (philosophy of life). Essentially, ethics offers a system of principles that assist in decision making.

Whilst undoubtedly fascinating, other texts are far better suited to portraying the history of ethics, and *A Short History of Ethics* (2002) by Alasdair MacIntyre covers an insightful history of moral philosophy from ancient to contemporary times. Whilst a detailed overview of ethics remains largely beyond the scope of the paramedic curriculum, this chapter will provide an overview of the different ethical branches within moral philosophy, as well as discussing applied ethics broadly within medicine. Ethical standpoints are outlined and the reader is encouraged to reflect upon and consider their own personal experiences and guiding actions towards developing a self-awareness of moral philosophy.

Normative Ethics

Normative (or prescriptive) ethics is concerned with developing a set of rules to govern human conduct. Looking to provide a set of norms for action, this branch of ethics is concerned with how things should be, what is good or bad (or right or wrong), and how to value actions and objects. Normative ethics are split into three main categories, which are as follows.

Consequentialism

Also known as teleological ethics, consequentialism argues that an action is judged whether it is ethically right or wrong by the consequences produced. An action is considered 'good' if, all things considered, the outcome or result is good. Therefore, in assessing the morality of an action, all of the good and all of the bad consequences must be weighed up. Similarly, if two different courses of action are presented, then the one chosen should have the best overall consequence. Any person who may be affected should be considered and one person's interests should not be considered over another's. From a utilitarian perspective, healthcare resources, finances and staffing are finite and should be appropriately accommodated to ensure society receives the best healthcare.

Consequentialism is an attractive theory – it seems difficult to argue that achieving the best outcome would be a bad thing. It relies on a similar style of reasoning when making purely practical decisions: when I am trying to decide how best to extricate the patient from the house, I will consider all the available options, judge the value of each option and then predict the option that will most likely lead to the best outcome: safe extrication and lack of manual handling for me. Using a mixture of personal and practical knowledge, I select the equipment. It is, fundamentally, a 'common-sense' approach.

However, the problem with consequentialism is defining 'good'. What is a 'good' method of extrication of a patient for me may not be a 'good' method for my crewmate. The most common consequentialist theory is *utilitarianism*. Coined by Jeremy Bentham, utilitarians claim that the most important good is for people to be happy – the greatest happiness for the greatest number. Therefore, in making ethical judgements, utilitarians ask which act will most increase the sum of human happiness. Some (referred to as *act utilitarians*) claim that the morality of each action is decided by which action, in certain or particular circumstances, is likely to promote the greatest happiness of the greatest number. Others (referred to as *rule utilitarians*) reject the idea that decisions should be based on circumstances and claim that it is the *type* of action that, if done by most people, promotes the greatest happiness of the greatest number. A good way to differentiate between act and rule utilitarianism is to consider the concept of lying. Suppose I tell my husband that I have put sugar in his tea, when really I haven't. Act utilitarians may consider that, in this particular case, this 'porky pie' is justified because it maximises the happiness of all those concerned (my husband thinks he is having sugar in his tea and I don't need to worry about him getting fat). However, a rule utilitarian would claim that since everyone lying would diminish happiness (my husband would be upset that there was no sugar in the tea and I would be upset if we argued about it), it would be best to adopt a rule against lying, even if in some cases telling a 'porky pie' may appear to promote the greatest good for the greatest number.

This raises another problem of consequentialism: 'good' for whom? Not putting sugar in tea is good for the waistline but not good if you like the taste of sweet tea! More seriously, what about when deciding about treatment for multiple patients at a large incident – is it only a question of what is best for one patient or best for all patients at that scene? Once every conceivable consequence of an action is considered, the decision-making process becomes much more complex.

This is not helped by the fact that we cannot predict what the consequences of our acts are (Smart 1993). If the consequences are so unpredictable, can we really use them as a guide to assess the morality of actions? Much of this is values-based, and *preference utilitarianism* allows individuals to be judged according to their own values (Singer 1994). *Teleology* also provides a moral basis for the professional ethics of medicine, as clinicians are generally concerned with outcomes and must therefore know the *telos* (the end goal) of a given treatment paradigm.

Other consequentialist theories hold different values at the centre of the ideology:

- *Altruism* – prescribes that individuals should take actions that have the best consequences for everyone, except for themselves. Its core tenet is a moral obligation to serve others and if necessary by sacrificing self-interest.

- *Asceticism* – describes a life lived abstaining from egoistical pleasures in order to achieve a spiritual goal.

- *Egoism* – holds that an action is right if it maximises good for the self; acting in one's own self-interest.

- *Hedonism* – holds that pleasure is at the centre of the pursuit of humankind and that individuals should strive to maximise their own pleasure (but not at the consequence of any pain or suffering).

Deontology

Deontology holds that our actions (or moral obligations) – whatever they may be – are independent of the consequences they produce. An action is good because it is right in itself. Going back to my earlier example, deontology would advocate that we should tell the truth not because it makes people happy or gives them pleasure, but because truth-telling is the *right* thing to do. The paramedic–patient relationship is, by nature, deontological and duty-bound.

Immanuel Kant is perhaps the best advocate of this maxim; his writings inspired Kantian ethics, a deontological ethical framework. Kant's *Universal Formula* posited the categorical imperative to 'Act in accordance with that maxim which can at the same time make itself into universal law' (Wood 2008: 82–83) and this is one of the central tenets of this theory. Kant advocated that no individual should be treated as a means to an end – a person should not be used merely to help others. Central to Kant's version of deontology is personhood: a moral person must construct their own moral law, which guides their actions. It is the ideal that one should treat others as one wishes to be treated themselves. Such principles may be demonstrated within medical research, where someone should not be used in research without their consent, even if that person may contribute to 'good' (for example, finding a cure for cancer). Clarity is often claimed as a deontological approach: if there is a clear deontological principle (such as not treating a patient without consent), then no further guidance is required. This is one reason why deontology is so attractive.

However, there are disagreements, and these generally centre around what the principles of good and bad behaviour are. Those with a religious faith may argue that what is good or bad is set by their God; those without may argue that some principles are naturally right or wrong. Principles such as truth, honesty and knowledge are considered 'self-evident', but in an increasingly multi-cultural, multi-faith and non-binary society, determining a social contract under which moral principles should be ranked is increasingly difficult.

In a similar way to consequentialism, those who hold deontological viewpoints may be split. Some deontologists argue that all deontological principles are absolute and cannot be breached under any circumstances. Others deviate from Kant's view that there should be a *Universal Formula* and may accept that if there are overwhelmingly good consequences, a breach may be justified (Morrison 2005). Consider the community first responder who breaks the speed limit to attend to a patient in cardiac arrest. Some would argue that the Highway Code should not be broken unless by a trained advanced driver. Others will accept that if there are overwhelmingly good consequences, a breach of the Highway Code may be justified. So, although a community first responder should not normally exceed the speed limit, some deontologists would argue that it may be appropriate to do so if they may save a life.

Generally, deontology is seen as an important response to consequentialism. Deontology aligns more with many concepts of human rights, although Kant places more emphasis on obligations than on rights. He describes humanity as having 'absolute and objective worth' as an end in itself, and the dignity of rational nature as an 'inner worth' that is 'beyond all price' (Wood 2008: 59). It is for this reason that many deontologists are against euthanasia; humans have intrinsic dignity and there is a universal law against killing. However, the distinction is not always clear. Whilst deontology may regard the consequences of an action to be irrelevant (for example, ignoring the importance of medical treatment), consequentialism may permit a paramedic to treat a patient without the patient's consent if the overall consequences of treatment were beneficial.

Essentially, these are perspectives and two different approaches to a problem, and sometimes clearer guidance is needed.

Virtue Ethics

Clearer guidance is not offered by virtue ethics. Virtue ethics is highly philosophical and emphasises the virtues (moral character), in contrast to the approach that emphasises the consequences of actions (consequentialism) or emphasises duties or rules (deontology). Essentially, virtue ethics focuses on the inherent character of the person rather than their actions or the nature of their consequences. This strand of ethics holds that a virtue is an excellent trait of character. It is a disposition – something intrinsic and deep in its possessor – to notice, expect, value, feel, desire, choose, act and react in certain characteristic ways (Rachels 1999). Virtue ethicists hold that is these behaviours that allow a person to achieve a good life (virtues) and guide the ability to achieve

Pause for Thought: The Trolley Problem

Imagine you are standing on a footbridge above tram tracks. You can see the runaway trolley (tram) hurtling towards five unsuspecting track workers, who cannot hear it coming. Even if they do spot it, they wouldn't be able to move away in time.

However, there is a morbidly obese man standing next to you on the footbridge. You're confident that his bulk would stop the tram in its tracks.

So, would you push the man on to the tracks, sacrificing him in order to stop the tram and thereby saving the five workers?

This is the crux of the classic thought experiment known as the trolley problem, developed by the philosopher Philippa Foot in 1967 and adapted by Judith Jarvis Thomson in 1985.

The trolley problem allows us to think through the consequences of an action and consider whether its moral value is determined solely by its outcome, and is a good way to illustrate the differences between utilitarianism and deontology. In the case of this dilemma, a utilitarian may advocate pushing the fat man and causing his death, but saving five others – thereby the fat man would be used as a means to an end.

There are lots of other thought-provoking examples of the trolley problem and they are well worth a review to help you determine your own ethical standpoint.

happiness. To possess a virtue is to be a certain sort of person with a certain complex mindset, and a significant aspect of this mindset is the wholehearted acceptance of a distinctive range of considerations as reasons for action.

Let us think back to our example about lying. In virtue ethics, an honest person is not simply someone who is honest; the motivation behind the action is important. Honesty should not be out of fear of being caught out or the outlook that 'honesty is the best policy', but related to a strong reason for not making false statements or actions. A virtue ethicist gives an overriding weight to 'truth' as the reason against dishonesty. Virtues are good habits that direct human nature towards good actions (Herring 2016). Within healthcare, the *6 Cs* were given in the Francis Report, which highlighted many examples of appalling care at the Mid Staffordshire Hospital in 2013. Jane Cummings, England's Chief Nursing Officer, launched the 6Cs strategy, which set out the shared purpose of nurses, midwives and health visitors against the backdrop of the Francis Inquiry. However, the strategy is not only limited to nursing and midwifery, having been adopted effectively across the NHS in the subsequent years. We therefore expect health professionals to act compassionately and competently, with care and commitment, as well as conducting good communication and having the courage to speak up when things go wrong. Whilst these are attractive principles and without doubt underpin the virtues health professionals should possess, in the heat of the moment, should the professional be confident that their decision was based on compassion and kindness or confident that the right course of action was chosen?

Ethics of Care

Virtue ethics is largely routed in Plato and Aristotle, who defined that the right action was the one that led to 'well-being' and can be achieved by a lifetime of practising virtues subject to practical wisdom. More recently, the ethics of care has been developed by feminist (a doctrine advocating social, political and all other rights for equality) writers and hold that moral action centres on interpersonal relationships and care, as well as benevolence as a virtue. Ethics of care avoid abstract tools and seek to find an approach that fits within individual cases (Tronto 1993).

One of the biggest criticisms is that the notion of care is too vague. Without a clear concept of what 'good' care is, it arguably should not form the basis of an ethical approach. Not all caring relationships are good ones, and problems with power and respect highlight the problems of this approach (Twigg 2000). Care should be explained in relational terms, in order not only to promote caring relationships, but also to explain that respect is central to good care.

Respect is also central to the universal vulnerability thesis, which outlines that everyone is vulnerable. The law has traditionally assumed people are self-sufficient and autonomous, and therefore individuals who do not fit into these categories are labelled as vulnerable. This approach indicates that our own health and well-being relies on that of others, and so the law should recognise society's mutual interdependence (Wrigley 2015). Ethics of care and moral philosophy overlap in several ways, and to understand more about this complex subject, I would recommend Virginia Held's *The Ethics of Care: Personal, Political, and Global* (2006).

Feminist Medical Ethics

What makes an ethical approach feminist? Is it because I am a female author that I have included this section? The feminist approach 'takes gender and sex as centrally important analytic categories, seeks to understand their operation in the world, and strives to change the distribution and use of power to stop the oppression of women' (Purdy 1996).

Feminist ethicists have worked to develop approaches to medical ethics that challenge how morality and virtues historically exemplified by women, such as patience, nurturing and self-sacrifice, are viewed. Such challenges are influential within the ethics of care (discussed above) and are also used to identify the inequalities in healthcare provision. Feminist work has highlighted disparities in gender health research (Scambler 2008), disproportionate gender views (Purdy 1996) and ignorance in the medical justification for the treatment of women (Lupton 1994).

Feminist ethics seeks to overcome the abstract theories applied by traditional medical ethics to complex clinical cases in order to understand the realities of individuals and their relation to the case overall (Marway and Widdows 2015). Perhaps we should pay more attention to this view going forward.

Hermeneutics

In its simplest form, hermeneutics is based on listening. It encourages the use of 'stories' and narratives, with the aim that listening brings about a shared understanding of the situation (Boyd 2005). Therefore, it offers an approach that does not suggest which are the right answers, but more what is right for those involved. This strand of ethics is central to the patient consultation, where the paramedic and the patient discuss a course of treatment. It seems somewhat idealistic that such a conversation can occur without the impact of other factors (such as fatigue) and requires a willingness to engage from all parties. However, where engagement does occur, this approach may enable the development of a solution that is tailored specifically to meet the needs of those involved.

Meta-ethics

A meta-ethical theory, unlike the normative ethical theories we have discussed, does not attempt to evaluate specific choices as being better or worse or good or bad; rather, it tries to define the essential meaning and nature of the problem being discussed. With 'meta' meaning above or beyond, meta-ethics consequently offers a 'bird's-eye view' of ethical concepts. It is concerned primarily with the *meaning* of ethical judgements and seeks to understand the nature of these judgements and how they may be defended or disputed. It concerns itself with questions specifically around the semantics, epistemology and ontology of ethics. It is highly theoretical and perhaps the least obviously applied to clinical practice. However, it is an important proponent for those undertaking, or wishing to undertake, further education or research.

Meta-ethics is a complex area and there are two main schools of thought within it. Whilst these may be broken down into further forms of their respected subjects, this chapter will deal with the overarching themes as an introduction.

Moral Realism

Moral realists hold that moral judgements describe moral facts, which are as accurate as mathematical or scientific facts. Moral realism is the view that moral facts and moral values exist independently of one's own perception of them, or their attitudes, beliefs or feelings towards them. Ethical sentences are therefore 'truth-apt' (they can be true or false) in their description of the real world. Some moral realist ethicists argue that an action should be taken at face value. If I have told my husband that I have put sugar in the tea, then I have. Moral claims imply that the facts reported are correct. In this way, moral realism allows straightforward logic to be applied to moral statements – so we could say that a moral belief is true in the same way that we would say this about a factual belief. However, some critics argue that the moral fact posited by this strand of ethics is non-material and therefore not accessible to the scientific method – in other words, that moral realism cannot replace observable science.

However, one advantage of moral realism is that this outlook allows moral conflict to be resolved: if two moral beliefs contradict each other, moral realism implies that they cannot both be right and therefore the situation may be resolved.

Moral Anti-realism

On the other hand, moral anti-realism holds that there are no objective moral values and is further split into the following:

- Ethical subjectivism – where any ethical sentence implies an attitude, opinion, personal preference or feeling held by someone.

- Non-cognitivism - where moral knowledge is impossible as ethical claims are neither true nor false and thereby do not express genuine propositions.

- Moral nihilism – where ethical claims are generally false and there are no objective moral values because there are no objective moral truths (an example being that a murder is neither wrong nor right).

Garner and Rosen provide an excellent summary on major topics within moral philosophy in their book *Moral Philosophy: A Systematic Introduction to Ethics and Meta-ethics*, and Alexander Miller presents not only a contemporary but also an applied view of meta-ethics in his *Contemporary Metaethics: An Introduction*. Both of these books provide a substantial overview to understanding the complex principles concerning meta-ethics and are recommended for those wishing to pursue this somewhat thorny subject further.

Descriptive Ethics

The branch of descriptive ethics examines ethics from the perspectives of the actual choice made by people in practice. It is value-free and, rather than prescribing theories of conduct or values, it looks at beliefs surrounding morality. Unlike normative ethics, it does not look to provide a guidance in making moral decisions, nor does it evaluate the reasonableness of ethical norms like meta-ethics. Instead, it is often used to compare ethical systems (between past and present, one society and another, or the ethics people claim to follow and the actual conduct of their actions). It is incredibly popular within the social sciences, including education, sociology, anthropology and history, although it still has a place in psychology and biology.

Applied Ethics

As the name suggests, applied ethics is the discipline of philosophy that attempts to apply ethical theory to real-life situations. An ethical dilemma arises when two or more courses of conduct may be justified in a given circumstance – what then is the right thing to do? The approaches to ethics already portrayed can often be strict and principle-based without giving solutions to specific problems, and as such may not be acceptable or applicable to implement. The discipline of applied ethics overcomes this by using a mixture of sociological and psychological insights to deliberate certain situations. Of all the branches of ethics already discussed, it is the most frequently used in determining public policy. Since this is a book aimed at paramedics, it is perhaps most obvious that our focus is on medical ethics. The legal, media, information, environmental and business sectors all have their own ethical principles and moral problems, but these are beyond the scope of what we present here.

Bioethics

The field of bioethics concerns the controversies brought about by advances and research in biology and medicine. Chapter 15 discusses some of the historical context that has shaped ethics in research, but with ongoing technical development, bioethics remains a fast-paced and professional area of inquiry.

Perhaps the most influential book concerning bioethics is *Principles of Biomedical Ethics* by Tom Beauchamp and James Childress (2013). This book advocates *Principlism*, so called because it is based on a set of principles that can be applied to any bioethical issue. They advocate four principles that represent a common morality (2013) across global cultures and that can be applied in a wide range of practical contexts. With uptake of this framework underpinning a variety of disciplinary teachings on medical ethics, these principles also ensure consistency in identifying moral issues in practice. Whilst they do not provide right or wrong answers to ethical issues, these principles allow clinicians to approach an issue flexibly, and enable clinicians and ethicists to balance these different principles in order to come to an agreement about a problem.

Beneficence

Beneficence is the principle that medical professionals must do good for their patients. This resonates within the Health and Care Professions Council (HCPC) Standards of Proficiency for paramedics to 'understand the need to act in the best interests of service users at all times' (HCPC 2016: 9). Across the medical disciplines, as well as within the military and the law, professionals are expected to put the needs of their service user first, even if it involves self-sacrifice (Downie 1988). This seems somewhat altruistic in a set of principles that do not align with any particular branch of ethics.

However, this principle focuses on the positive ethical obligations applied within the medical context and deals with seeking to benefit others. This concept is central to most people's ethical thinking and remains a central pillar in the practice of medical ethics.

Non-maleficence

Non-maleficence is the principle that one person should not cause harm to others. It is best understood that, as a whole, a medical intervention should not cause harm. Evidently, most attempts to benefit a patient require the infliction of harm or involve risks of harm. Inserting a cannula or performing a needle chest decompression are good examples of this. Taking non-maleficence literally would lead the clinician to do nothing at all.

Therefore, this is often taken as balancing the principle of beneficence (a clinician's obligation to help a patient) against the obligation not to cause harm.

There is also a wide-ranging understanding of harms. The concept of harm is inextricably bound to human vulnerability and, as such, Harrosh (2011: 494) outlines four modes of human vulnerability which may cause harm:

- As conscious beings, negative experiences including (but not limited to) pain, discomfort, disappointment, irritations, sadness, anxiety and humiliation can be harmful.

- The presence of disease and the improper functioning of the body's systems, organs, cognitions or emotions can harm the physical and psychological integrity of what makes someone human.

- Interests formed as rational human beings can leave us vulnerable to harm if we experience setbacks or if the goals and values of our lives are compromised.

- To enable a fully human life, we can be harmed if we do not have the opportunity to engage with the basic goods of life, such as relationships, and experience connectedness with others.

It is worth noting that these are not mutually exclusive and nor is this list exhaustive. Nevertheless, this presents an idea of the different ways in which humans can be harmed, and therefore different ways in which maleficence can occur. In order to act in a truly non-maleficent way, clinicians should bear in mind the varying guises under which harm may occur in order to ensure a profession free from it.

Autonomy

The principle of autonomy is the respect given to individuals as independent moral agents, with the right to choose how to live their own lives. It is seen as a fundamental aspect of humanity and is one of the individual rights under the European Convention on Human Rights (ECHR) and protected by law. 'To respect autonomy is to accept a person has the right to hold views, make choices and take actions based on personal values and beliefs' (Herring 2016: 28). This principle is slightly deontological in its approach – discarding a person's wishes or beliefs would mean that people are treated as a means to an end, the opposite of what Kant advocated.

It is important to outline that the patient does not have the right to the type of medical treatment given or to demand specific treatments, such as cosmetic surgery. What is claimed is a right to bodily integrity – a right to not have something done to the body without consent. Equally, autonomy does not mean that every choice is respected, but only those that are competent. This book will later outline problems surrounding decisions made by children (see Chapter 11) and those suffering from mental ill-health (see Chapters 9 and 10).

However, care must be taken with competence – just because a person's decision may be considered foolish does not mean they are incompetent. A clinician may believe a patient's decision to be ill-advised, but the decision remains the patient's to make and must be respected. In many cases, following a patient's decision will be promoting their welfare. In others, if treatment is forced upon a patient against their will, then the patient will suffer. A common example of this is the patient who is a Jehovah's Witness, who refuses a blood transfusion even though without it, they will die. Autonomy is not respected because it promotes welfare rather than respecting their human rights (Molyneux 2009).

Justice

Justice is concerned with what is fair and reasonable – in healthcare, the distribution of resources, both financial and in terms of access to healthcare. The justice of health often looks to overcome issues apparent in healthcare inequality, where in many systems, certain ethnic groups or those of lower socioeconomic status suffer worse health than other groups (Bartley and Bane 2009). Such inequalities can present a major political issue and therefore the justice of health often relates to the politics of the time.

Central to the principle of justice is the theory of formal equality: everyone is equal. I particularly like what William Frankena (1962) said about this: 'all men are to be treated as equals, not because they are equal, in any respect, but simply because they are all human'. This principle is uncontroversial, but there seem to be broad problems with its application. For more on the application of social justice, I would recommend 'Displacing the Distributive Paradigm' by Iris Young (1997).

Medical Ethics

The field of medical ethics is the study of moral values and judgements as they are applied to the practice of medicine. As a profession allied to medicine, these moral values translate within all aspects of paramedic practice. Arguably, medical ethics should reflect the moral values that are regarded as acceptable amongst healthcare professionals, as well as society as a whole.

A Little History

Whilst MacIntyre covers the history of ethics beautifully, I wanted to pay homage to the development of ethics within medicine. Historically, Western medical ethics has been traced to guidelines concerning the duty of physicians, with initial outlines of this duty within the Hippocratic Oath. The Oath required a new physician to swear upon a number of healing gods that he would uphold the professional standards. It also bound the student physician to his teacher and the greater community of physicians. As well as being recognised as an early stage of medical training, the Oath was also the earliest expression of medical ethics in the Western hemisphere. The Oath has, in many contexts, allowed medicine to develop paternalistically – where the clinician acts for the benefit (and in the best interests) of another, without specific consent. Up until the last half-century, paternalism has meant patients have often been treated without adequate explanation of their illness or injury.

Sometimes caught up within the Hippocratic Oath is the saying 'First, do no harm' (or *Primum non nocere* if your Latin is up to scratch). Contrary to popular belief, this phrase was coined as recently as 1860 and is attributed to Thomas Inman (a house surgeon at Liverpool Royal Infirmary), and remains central to ethics in today's Western medicine. The perception of what constitutes harm will be different across service users, and the expected benefits will also be different. The limits to interpreting this phrase verbatim are similar to the discussion within non-maleficence, and the principles of beneficence and non-maleficence remain central to understanding this. Ultimately, these principles are best assessed in the principles respecting autonomy and justice (Sokol 2013).

Current Medical Ethics

The ideals of Principlism are adopted into a majority of medical systems and it provides a good example of how ethical discourse necessitates reflection and justification of our actions by reference to accepted morals and values (Gordon et al. 2011).

The state of current medical ethics is attributed to a tapestry interwoven with a range of philosophical theories (Laurie et al. 2016); however, out of all those discussed, deontology and utilitarianism continue to remain the most evident attitudes across the majority of healthcare settings. Nevertheless, different ethical paradigms are required for each healthcare setting – whilst deontology may still work in a clinician–patient relationship, public health focuses much more on a consequentialist approach. One set of principles that draws on both deontology and utilitarian thinking is communitarianism. *Communitarian ethics* emphasises both the obligations we owe to others (the deontological angle) and on the consequences of our individual decisions (consequentialism). It allows different values to simultaneously be at stake, responding to the clinical context involved.

However, the principle that has dominated medical law and ethics for the last 50 years remains being autonomous. This directly clashes with the historical paternalistic culture on the basis of which medicine (as well as paramedicine) has evolved, and has empowered the patient to be at the centre of medical care rather than just the recipient. Yet, there are warnings with the current empowerment of autonomy. Accepting individualistic autonomy as 'good' can lead to other values being disregarded and can have negative effects. There must be a social dimension to autonomy, and personal autonomy should be measured against the needs of society as a whole. Western society demands a just distribution of resources. Therefore, whilst in an ideal world a sick person should be able to demand the treatment of their choice, this choice is limited by the framework provided by the society in which they reside (Campbell 1994).

Rights theory also plays another important role in current medical ethics. Hearing patients say 'it's my right to have such-and-such' is a good example of how the language of rights has become combative and assertive, where it hinders rather than helps moral consensus. Rights do exist in ethics (and law), but misunderstanding has often boiled them down into declarations rather than the original intentions of principled behaviour. Rights talk often leads to a moral impasse, where neither the patient's rights nor the clinician's rights are taken into account. A confrontational declaration of rights is unlikely to be constructive in guiding decision making, but it should be remembered that the rights on both sides have the obligation to work towards the ideal.

Ethics and Law

The different branches of ethics create a particular problem for medical law: should the law be based on ethical principles? If so, which principles should be followed? In the Western hemisphere, Judeo-Christian values predominantly guide the law, with a strong emphasis on intrinsic human dignity. However, this is slowly being eroded and laws within a historical religious context are now being revoked, such as the availability of abortion.

The Eighth Amendment of the Constitution of Ireland

The Eighth Amendment of the Constitution Act 1983 amended the Constitution of Ireland by recognising the equal right to life of both the unborn fetus and the pregnant woman. Abortion had been subject to criminal penalty in Ireland since 1861 and the amendment ensured that abortion was only allowed in circumstances where the life of a pregnant woman was at risk. This was approved by a referendum on 7 September 1983 and was signed into law on 7 October 1983. The Campaign to Repeal the Eighth Amendment gained traction following an unsuccessful anti-amendment campaign in 1983, and on 25 May 2018, a referendum was conducted, in which voters overwhelmingly supported repealing the constitutional ban on abortion; this is currently awaiting being signed into law.

The Hippocratic Oath also sets out principles that have been adopted to form the foundation of ethics in medicine. Alongside autonomy (which is covered in both the Hippocratic Oath and in Principlism), two other principles seem to be particularly special, as they are also expressed as rights within medical law: the right to life and the right to dignity.

The right to life, the right of autonomy and the right to dignity are protected within individuals' rights under the ECHR (also known as the Convention for the Protection of Human Rights and Fundamental Freedoms), which sets out the minimum standard of treatment people are entitled to expect under the law. The ECHR is a 'living instrument', which means that its articles must be interpreted in the context of contemporary conditions. Societies and values change, and the Courts take account of these changes when interpreting the ECHR.

The human rights most frequently discussed in the context of medicine are:

- the right to life
- the right to health
- the right to autonomy
- the right to dignity
- the right to privacy
- the right to equality
- the right not to be tortured or subjected to cruel or inhuman treatment
- the right to bodily integrity.

However, this book focuses on three rights that are considered to be the most fundamental.

The Right to Life

For many people, the right to life is a key human right. It is also the cause of many disagreements within ethics, as well as within legal systems across different countries. Debate on the meaning of life and what it means to respect the right to life has particular implications in the context of euthanasia and abortion. In addition, the right to die is not incumbent. Article 2 of the ECHR protects the right of every person to their life.

The Right to Autonomy

Personal autonomy, protected by Article 8 of the ECHR, is the right to decide what medical treatment an individual receives. However, it is much more complex than merely deciding what treatment can be received, and more closely follows the right to refuse treatment. Conceptually, personal autonomy includes both the physical freedom to act as a free agent as well as the 'psychological sense', which is the freedom 'to know what we can do if we want to'. It also includes such matters as choosing how to spend one's final days and how to manage one's death. Whilst the focus is on the individual, the right to autonomy must not interfere with the rights of others, and a balance must be found between the interests of the individual and the public. The right to autonomy is often used in conjunction with the right to dignity.

The Right to Dignity

Dignity refers to what is special about an individual. The right to dignity is founded on a very Kantian outlook, where human dignity rests on autonomy (in the context of living under a universalisable law that self-legislating reason prescribes for itself, as opposed to making your own choices) which is inherent in each individual (Kass 2002: 16). The dignity interests protected by the ECHR include, under Article 3, the right to die with dignity and the right to be protected from treatment, or from a lack of treatment, which would result in someone dying in avoidably distressing circumstances. A failure to provide life-prolonging treatment in circumstances exposing the patient to 'inhuman or degrading treatment' would in principle involve a breach of Article 3. Even if the patient's suffering had not reached the level of severity required to breach Article 3, a withdrawal of treatment in the same circumstances might still breach Article 8 if there were sufficiently adverse effects on the patient's physical or moral integrity or mental stability.

Respecting a person's dignity requires far more than respecting their choices, and at the heart of the right to dignity is the concept that all humans have an intrinsic worth and that their moral agency should be respected (Neal 2012).

Summary

This chapter has presented an overview of ethics concerned with paramedic practice. The ethical principles outlined are applicable to clinical, research, education and leadership environments – indeed, any environment in which a paramedic may find themselves. Ethical dilemmas will exist when these theories or principles clash, but an awareness of the reader's own morals will ensure that any such clashes are acknowledged and can be dealt with in order to ensure the autonomy and best interests of all those concerned.

✳ Case Study

You are an advanced paramedic, working in a rural GP practice. Having recently finished your independent prescribing course, you have your own patient list as well as running a minor illness clinic three afternoons a week. In the middle of a busy clinic, you see a regular patient for the second time that day, who is now complaining of ankle pain following looking after a neighbour's chickens. The patient has some cuts to her lower legs and the right ankle is more bruised than the other, but there is no evidence of inflammation, despite the patient telling you so. You advise a soft tissue injury, with management following this approach. Four days later, you receive notification that this patient has been admitted to hospital with signs of sepsis. One day later, the practice is notified of the patient's death due to severe sepsis with organ dysfunction.

The patient's family immediately demand answers from the practice, knowing their relative saw you before they died. The practice manager is pressuring you to apologise in the hope of mitigating legal trouble. You are doubting your practice and are afraid that if you admit a mistake, you will be in trouble with both the practice and your regulatory body.

What do you do? Should you apologise and explain to the family what went wrong? What are the risks of doing so? Do you have an ethical obligation to admit error? What are the possible benefits to admitting fault? Is there anything the GP practice should have done differently? Was this a preventable mistake?

Recommended Reading

Garner, R and Rosen, B (1967) *Moral Philosophy: Systematic Introduction to Normative Ethics and Meta-ethics*. New York: Macmillan.

Glover, J (1990) *Causing Death and Saving Lives*. London: Penguin.

Harris, J (1985) *The Value of Life*. London: Routledge.

Held, V (2006) *The Ethics of Care: Personal, Political, and Global.* Oxford: Oxford University Press.

MacIntyre, A (2002) *A Short History of Ethics*. London: Routledge.

Young, M (1997) Displacing the distributive paradigm. In H LaFollette (ed), *Ethics in Practice: An Anthology.* Oxford: Blackwell: 547–58.

References

Bartley, M and Blane, D (2009) Inequality and social class. In G Scambler (ed), *Sociology as Applied to Medicine* (pp. 115–32). New York: Saunders.

Beauchamp, T and Childress, J (2013) *Principles of Biomedical Ethics*, 6th ed. Oxford: Oxford University Press.

Boyd, K (2005) Medical ethics: principles, persons and perspectives: from controversy to conversation. *Journal of Medical Ethics*, 31: 481–86.

Campbell, A (1994) Dependency: the foundational value in medical ethics. In KVM Fulford and GJM Gillet (eds), *Medicine and Moral Reasoning (*pp. 184–92). Cambridge: Cambridge University Press.

Downie, R (1988) Traditional medical ethics and economics in health care: a critique. In G Mooney and A McGuire (eds), *Medical Ethics and Economics in Health Care (pp. 40–55).* Oxford: Oxford University Press.

Frankena, W (1962) The Concept of Social Justice. In Brandt R (ed), *Social Justice*. New Jersey: Englewood Cliffs

Gillon, R (2012) When four principles are too many: a commentary. *Journal of Medical Ethics*, 38: 197–98.

Gordon, J-S, Rauprich, O and Vollmann, J (2011) Applying the four-principle approach. *Bioethics*, 25: 293–300.

Harrosh, S (2011) Identifying harms. *Bioethics Online*. Available at: https://doi.org/10.1111/j.1467-8519 .2011.01889.x.

Health and Care Professions Council (HCPC) (2016) *Standards of Proficency: Paramedics*. London: Health and Care Professions Council.

Herring, J (2016) *Medical Law and Ethics*, 6th ed. Oxford: Oxford University Press.

Kant, I (1997) *Groundwork for the Metaphysics of Morals, 1785,* M Gregor (trans). Cambridge: Cambridge University Press.

Kass, L (2002) *Life, Liberty and the Defence of Dignity: The Challenge for Bioethics*. San Francisco: Encounter Books.

Laurie, G, Harmon, S and Porter, G (2016) *Mason and McCall Smith's Law and Medical Ethics*. 10th ed. Oxford: Oxford University Press.

Lupton, D (1994) *Medicine as Culture*. London: Sage.

Marway, H and Widdows, H (2015) Philosophical Feminist Bioethics. *Cambridge Quarterly of Healthcare Ethics*, 24 (2): 165–74.

Molyneux, D (2009) Should healthcare professionals respect autonomy just because it promotes welfare? *Journal of Medical Ethics*, 35: 245–50.

Morrison, D (2005) A holistic approach to clinical and research decision-making. *Medical Law Review*, 13: 45–79.

Neal, M (2012) Not gods but animals: human dignity and vulnerable subjecthood. *Liverpool Law Review,* 33: 177–200.

Purdy, L (1996) A feminist view of health. In S Wolf (ed), *Feminism and Bioethics* (pp. 163–83). Oxford: Oxford University Press.

Rachels, J (1999) *The Elements of Moral Philosophy*. London: McGraw-Hill.

Scambler, A (2008) Women and health. In G Scambler (ed), *Sociology as Applied to Medicine* (pp. 133–58). London: Saunders.

Singer, P (1994) *Rethinking Life and Death*. Oxford: Oxford University Press

Smart, J (1993) *Utilitarianism: For and Against*. Cambridge: Cambridge University Press.

Sokol, DK (2013). "First do no harm" revisited. *BMJ*, 347(7932): 23.

Sommerville, A (2003) Juggling law, ethics, and intuition: practical answers to awkward questions. *Journal of Medical Ethics*, 29: 281–86.

Tronto, J (1993) *Moral Boundaries: A Political Argument for an Ethic of Care*. New York: Routledge.

Twigg, J (2000) Carework as a form of bodywork. *Ageing and Society*, 20: 389–411.

Wrigley, A (2015) An eliminativist approach to vulnerability. *Bioethics* 29(7): 478–487.

Wood, A (2008) *Kantian Ethics*. Cambridge: Cambridge University Press.

Chapter 4	An Overview of British Law
	Keiran Bellis

Introduction

Though the UK is a unitary state, it comprises three other legal systems followed in England and Wales, Scotland, and Northern Ireland, with the latter two also being influenced by the common law system in England (Wales started following the system from 1536). This chapter will discuss the legal frameworks that exist, including the historical underpinnings of today's legal system, and how laws are created, amended and applied in practice. This is a complex chapter, presenting the many complexities of the legal system and how these influence paramedic practice.

The English Legal System

Whilst development of the common law was promoted by the early dominant position acquired by the royal courts, depending on who held power, the signing of the Magna Carta in 1215 heralded the dawn of the English legal system. This has subsequently developed and evolved into the current system today, which, unlike many others within the Western world, is not rooted within a written constitution. Despite there being no formal written constitution, there is a widespread acceptance that we do in fact follow a set of rules. These amount to an informal constitution, as many aspects of law development, creation and implementation are culminated within a written Bill of Rights, which sets out certain basic civil rights. One of the key elements that underpin this model is the legal separation of powers that distinguishes between the executive, legislature and judicial arms of the country. Within this legal framework, we would consider the government to be the executive, Parliament to be the legislature and the judicial element being executed by judges within the judiciary. The basis of this theory is that the three arms of the power, or the basis of power, should not be held by one person or group, but that a system is in place for ratification and conferment of any decisions made.

A second fundamental principle of the English domestic legal system is the notion that Parliament holds supremacy and is the highest source of English law as long as the law has been passed in accordance with the rules of parliamentary procedure. This is also referred to as parliamentary sovereignty. In explaining this, Dicey (1982, pp. 3–4) famously commented that according to the principle of supremacy, Parliament has 'the right to make or unmake any law whatsoever; and further, no person or body is recognised by law in England as having the right to override or set aside the legislation of Parliament'. One ongoing challenge to this concept, and what many commentators note as an erosion of parliamentary supremacy, is Britain's current relationship with the European Union (EU). Whilst the EU can only develop legislation in certain subject areas, there is an expectation for domestic law to be set aside, and EU law takes precedence over domestic law.

A final basic principle of English law is the rule of law, this being that there should be no sanction without a breach; put simply, no person should be punished by the state unless they have broken a law. A second aspect of the rule of law is that one law should govern us all, whether that is the man on the Clapham omnibus, a state official or a paramedic discharging their duty. Finally, the last aspect is that the rights of individuals should be protected by the judiciary rather than by Parliament or any constitutional body.

Northern Ireland, Scotland and Wales

In 1998, a number of important constitutional changes were made as a result of the passing of the Scotland Act 1998, the Northern Ireland Act 1998 and the Government of Wales Act 1998. This led to the creation of the Scottish Parliament, and the Northern Ireland and Welsh Assemblies respectively, and within this devolution, some law-making powers have been devolved to the home countries.

The new Scottish Parliament, created by the Scotland Act 1998, can make laws affecting Scotland only, on many important areas, including health, education, local government, criminal justice, food standards and agriculture. However, legislation on foreign affairs, defence, national security, trade, industry and a number of other areas are still made for the whole of the UK by the Westminster Parliament.

Similarly, the Northern Ireland Act 1998 gives the Northern Ireland Assembly the power to make legislation for Northern Ireland in some areas, though again, foreign policy, defence and certain other areas are still to be covered by Westminster.

In the same year, the Government of Wales Act 1998 established a new body for Wales: the Welsh Assembly. Like the other two bodies, the Welsh Assembly has the power to make primary legislation on subject areas where power has been devolved; otherwise, legislation made in Westminster will continue to cover Wales regarding policing, justice, social security and most areas of commercial/business law. However, the Welsh Assembly is able to make what is called delegated legislation. This is a subsection of legislation designed to affect only those within a particular region, such as Highway Orders and matters relating to the cost of higher education. England and Wales still have a very harmonious legal system as the vast majority of laws emanating from Parliament are passed with the intention of covering both countries.

Sources of Law

Whilst much of the law today is built through case law or common law, it is actually statute law or an Act of Parliament which is commonly considered to hold the greatest legal importance within domestic law. In addition to statute law and common law, the English legal system is also framed to a significant degree around EU law. These are the three most likely sources of law that will influence paramedic practice, though laws can also be developed through delegated legislation, often council by-laws, international treaties and occasionally accepted customs within a country or territory.

Statute Law

One of the complexities of understanding the law is getting to grips with the language. Statute law and Acts of Parliament are terms which are used interchangeably. They both have the same meaning in essence as the law or act passes through the parliamentary process. This process is set out in Figure 4.1, which shows the degree of scrutiny that is entrenched within the separation of powers as a bill passes through the House of Commons three times, before passing through the House of Lords, before being presented to the monarch for Royal Assent, before being applied by the judiciary in the courts. It's a complicated process!

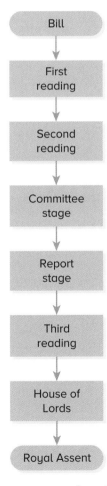

Figure 4.1 The passage of an Act of Parliament

The actual application of the law is the domain of the courts. Reaching overall agreement on all the events resulting from every Act of Parliament has proven challenging over the years, and this is partly the reason why a common law system is required to support the statutory provision. In an ideal world, there would be legislative and parliamentary certainty surrounding all acts, but this is not realistically possible and, as a consequence, the courts will look to a number of sources for guidance when applying the law relating to the case before them. Whilst the intention of Parliament should be explicit within the wording of the Act, Bennion (2005) highlighted a number of possible reasons why the true intention of the Act may be ambiguous and lead to judicial uncertainty. These ambiguities arise when, during the drafting of the legislation, words are omitted or considered to be implied. A further issue noted by Bennion (2005) is that broad terms are used to try to capture the essence of the law, but this serves to add some confusion. A good example is using the term 'motor vehicles' instead of cars, vans or any other prohibited vehicles. General ambiguity is a common factor in many pieces of legislation, highlighted by the European Communities Act 1972, in relation to how the UK applied EU law.

English Law Rules for Statutory Interpretation

In English law, there are three rules that exist to assist a court in the interpretation of an Act of Parliament. These rules are the most common approach in examining the meaning of the language used or the application to which the statute was intended, or a combination of both.

The Literal Rule

The literal rule takes precedence over the others and states that the words in the statute must be interpreted to mean exactly what they say, however absurd or unfair the conclusion.

Within this, the meaning of the word must be determined by its context and any general term is dependent on any specific terms that precede it.

The Golden Rule

The golden rule tells the reader of the statute to read the word in the context of the sentence as a whole and tries to assess what it was that Parliament was trying to do when writing it. This can be applied in two ways: first, if there is ambiguity in the meaning of several words, then preference is given to the word which does not result in absurdity; and, second, this rule can be used to modify a word that has only one meaning in order to avoid an absurd outcome.

The Mischief Rule

This rule attempts to determine the legislator's intention and is primarily used to interpret a statute that was passed in order to remedy a common law loophole (also known as mischief). This rule is used by the courts to decide what loophole the statute was intended to correct or close. In doing so, the courts go beyond the words of the statute to ascertain what loophole the statute was set out to remedy.

The key factor within the application of statute law is for the judiciary to ascertain what exactly Parliament had intended to be covered within the act. This notion of parliamentary intention should create a degree of certainty, but as these problems are often discussed tens (or sometimes hundreds) of years after each law was created, there is no way of going back to ask Parliament what it was that was truly intended. This is where the common law system seeks to fill the gaps, though as seen in the *Cusack v London Borough of Harrow* (2013) case, the Supreme Court felt that any guidance to support the interpretation of statutes should be seen as 'guidelines rather than railway lines'. Within this case, it was argued that often statute law provides legislative certainty due to the difficult and long path to amend or change Acts of Parliament, though this is often returned as a criticism as it is seen as inflexible and not necessarily all-encompassing. It is often these criticisms which highlight why the English legal system is not solely based upon acts as written, and so additional legal systems are required, such as case law.

Pause for thought

Taking a very simple example for paramedics, for instance cannulation. If the use of cannulation was to have been restricted in an Act after the introduction of Paramedics in the 1990s, should that restriction be applied to interosseous infusion in 2018? What was the intention of Parliament when restricting the use of intravenous access equipment and did they or could they have foreseen alternative tools for gaining vascular access when the law was hypothetically drafted?

Case Law

Case law, or common law as it is often referred to, is the oldest legal system within England dating back to the Norman invasion (1066). The common law system drew together the many regional courts in an attempt to standardise the law across the country and by 1250, a 'common law' had been produced. From the notion of *stare decisis,* judges now follow decisions made in the higher courts, and it is this system of precedent and case law that exists within the courts of the twenty-first century. A case law system does not escape criticism, as many black letter lawyers (a very traditional perspective rooted in the strict application of law as it is written) feel that a legal system is being created where the judiciary are creating law rather than merely applying it. Such claims of judge-made law were countered by Blackstone in 1765, who stated that 'judges do not make law, but merely, by the rules of precedent, discover and declare the law that has always been'. If a bad decision is made, a new one can be made to reverse this. This is not a new law, but merely a correct interpretation of the current provision. He further noted that the judges' decisions were not based upon personal thoughts and feelings, but known laws and customs of the land. This notion is a little troublesome in practice, as many

> *Stare decisis is Latin for "to stand by things decided." In short, it is the doctrine of precedent. Courts cite to stare decisis when an issue has been previously brought to the court and a ruling already issued.*

judges over many years have been known to be more conservative and less liberal, and vice versa.

The development of the body of case law comes from cases with judicial precedent from previous cases with similar facts to the case in hand. When this is presented, the courts are bound to apply the principles found in the case from a higher court, which is known as following the previous judgment. The problems arise when this is not entirely possible and there are three other options available to the judge in this instance:

1. They can choose to distinguish the facts from the previous case, which is that the facts are significantly different from those in the earlier case and thus they are no longer bound by its decision.

2. The judge may overrule the decision. If the decision is one from a lower court, this is effectively set aside and no longer followed (although this is actioned infrequently as it could be seen as weakening the powers of the lower courts).

3. The court may choose to overrule a previous decision, which is common practice. Although this may be oversimplifying the process, typically decisions are more complex than just overruling one case and there are often numerous case decisions considered within each new case. This can be demonstrated in the *Montgomery v Lanarkshire* case (2015), which appears to have overruled the test for informed consent created by McNair J in *Bolam v Friern Hospital Management Committee* (1957) (the Bolam test), which was later affirmed (and then discounted) in the *Sidaway* case.

Sidaway Board of Governors of Bethlem Royal Hospital and Others (1985)

Mrs Sidaway suffered from chronic pain in her neck, right shoulder and arm, and consented to a spinal cord decompression. Her neurosurgeon explained the procedure, but did not warn of all the side-effects, specifically that in less than 1% of all spinal cord decompression attempts, there is a risk of paraplegia. As a consequence of the operation, she became paralysed.

In rejecting her claim for damages, the court stated that in order to obtain consent, it was not required for the doctors to give an elaborate explanation of the remote side-effects of the procedure. The court adopted the principles as laid out in the Bolam test to support this position.

Case law relating directly to ambulance practice is rather scarce, as it is the principles that need to be applied rather than the facts of the precedent that are key. However, there is one seminal case that demonstrated the ambulance service's duty of care to its patients and highlighted a number of the principles which have already been discussed. *Kent v Griffiths* (2000) established a duty of care for the ambulance service when accepting an emergency call and a duty to respond in an appropriate timeframe. The judge considered the duty of care of the emergency services to respond to incidents, but the basis of that statutory duty differs between the emergency services. One further point that must be considered is that judges, rather than juries, set precedents. Therefore, it is the prerogative of the higher courts to develop the common law system.

The Civil and Criminal Law Pathways

When many people first think about the law and legal issues, it is often the criminal courts that initially spring to mind, despite there being a significantly lower incidence of criminal law involvement within healthcare law fields than is seen in the civil courts. The two court systems are very distinct and rarely cross paths. Despite both originating in the magistrates' court and then both utilising the same higher courts, the rules applied and the language used in both tracks are extremely different. The civil courts see actions, litigation or 'being sued', whereas in a criminal court, the defendant is prosecuted. The burden of proof within each court is different too, with civil cases being decided on the balance of probabilities, that being a 51% certainty that the alleged action led to the wrong being claimed. This differs vastly from that within a criminal court, where the burden of proof is beyond all reasonable doubt, thus being as close to 100% sure as you can be. This is a cornerstone of our criminal justice system and ensures that the state can have the utmost confidence in its convictions, though this has been shown to be flawed from time to time. Another facet of the English criminal law system is that no person leaves the courtroom innocent; they are merely not guilty. This may appear to be semantics, but there is a key difference in the two notions. Civil acts can be viewed as unlawful, whereas criminal acts are illegal. There are no specific criteria that make an act a criminal offence or a civil wrong, except those laid out in the law, and some events can be both criminal and civil wrongs. Imagine you are driving to an emergency using your visual and audible warning devices, but travelling at 60 mph in a 30 mph zone. You collide with a vehicle when passing through a red light and unfortunately kill a passenger in the other vehicle. This might result in you being prosecuted by the state, contrary to section 1 of the Road Traffic Act 1991, for causing death by dangerous driving, which is a criminal offence. You may also be sued by the deceased's family for negligence as each time a driver takes to the road, they have an established duty of care to drive safely and in accordance with the law. Any driving exemption that might be claimed in emergency driving does not negate any negligence. The semantics continue with the overall tone of prosecution and guilt in the criminal courts, and action and liability in the civil courts.

However, many cases in this area are brought against the employer rather than the individual. This is done under the doctrine of vicarious liability. This doctrine imposes a liability on employers when the wrong (or tort) occurs in the normal discharge of their duties – for example, a paramedic acting within their own scope of practice and not maliciously inflicting harm upon a patient. Compare this with a paramedic who attempts to insert a chest drain or perform a finger thoracotomy without the education to support such advanced practice, or the Emergency Medical Technician who chooses to cannulate a patient and administer a drug. Even if these clinicians can provide a defence or rationale, the court is unlikely to support a notion of vicarious liability. The basis for this position emanates from two key cases concerning bus operators in London in the mid-nineteenth century and at the turn of the twentieth century, *Limpus v London General Omnibus Company* (1861) and *Beard v London General Omnibus Company* (1900). The facts of these cases are set out below.

Limpus v London General Omnibus Company (1861)

A driver of an omnibus pulled out across the path of an omnibus from a rival company to try to get ahead of his rival. He did this despite being issued with a card requesting him not to race with or obstruct another omnibus.

The matter for the court to decide was whether the act was undertaken for the purpose of his employer or if it was an act of his own. The court found that the employer was liable for the accident as it was an act done in the course of his duty as a bus driver. This meant the London General Omnibus Company holding vicarious liability for a negligent act completed by an employee.

Beard v London Omnibus Company (1900)

In order to save time at the terminus, a conductor employed by the London Omnibus Company chose to drive the bus around to prepare it for his return journey. During this, the bus struck Mr Beard, negligently causing an injury.

Mr Beard attempted to sue the bus company, but failed in his action, as the court noted that he had failed to provide any evidence that the conductor had been authorised to drive the bus and therefore had failed to establish that the company should be held vicariously liable for the individual's negligent acts.

The Civil Courts

Civil cases are usually between two parties and typically do not have any state involvement. This is certainly true in the lower courts, but in many high-profile cases, the state does become involved in appeals within the higher courts. The lack of state involvement is seen as a key facet of England's civil court structure: aside from providing the courts and the personnel, it was intended that the state should not interfere in private hearings. The state involvement within the higher courts arises from appeals where the Crown or 'R' acts on behalf of one of the parties. The Crown can be a plaintiff or a defendant in civil actions. Civil actions have a very specific language which has very subtle variations depending on the circumstances in which the case is being heard. Within the courts of first instance, the county court, the magistrate's court and the High Court, the parties in each case are the the claimant and the person whom the action is being brought against is the defendant. If or when the case moves to the Court of Appeal, the parties are then referred to as the appellant and the respondent. As a result of the Civil Procedure Rules (1998), which came about directly as a result of the passing of the Civil Procedure Act 1997, three paths of litigation were created. These are referred to as tracks, with the small claims track, the fast track and the multi-track. There are a number of key determinants as to which claims track a claimant will need to pursue and these are based largely upon the value of the claim. The small claims track can be utilised for debt claims of up to £10,000 or personal injury claims of up to £1,000 and these cases will be heard in the county court. The next stage within this process is the fast track; this allows for claims of up to £25,000 to be heard within the county court, but if the case is classed as complex, it may escalate to the High Court if required. Finally, there is the multi-track: due to the cost of these claims, it is likely this would be passed to the High Court for trial, though these cases can also be heard in the county court. Despite the guidance set down in the Civil Procedure Rules, a *Practice Direction* (1991) has indicated that there are a number of types of action which must be heard in the High Court. These include cases involving professional negligence and fatal accidents, defamation, fraud and false imprisonment, amongst others. Negligence is the most likely claim against a clinician and this will be discussed in greater depth in Chapter 8. Whilst most cases start within the county court system, the magistrates' court plays a role in the civil law process, where it has powers of recovery for utilities and council tax, as well as presiding over licences to sell alcohol. All of these are seen as civil processes, though the consequences for non-payment may then involve the criminal courts.

The High Court, the Court of Appeal and the Supreme Court

The High Court of Justice was created in 1873. The lead civil division is currently the Queen's Bench Division, the others being the Family Division (dealing with family issues) and the Chancery Division, which deals primarily with business law, trust and probate-type cases. All cases that are tortious in nature (negligence, breach of duty of care and similar wrongs) will be heard by this court. Decisions of the High Court can be appealed to the Court of Appeal (Civil Division), where the case will typically be heard by three senior judges, though this can be as many as five in very important cases and as little as two in interim appeals. The *Kent v Griffiths* (2000) case was heard in the Court of Appeal. The London Ambulance Service had argued that it should not be liable for damages awarded by the High Court; its appeal failed and all three judges agreed that it was 'reasonably foreseeable' that the claimant would suffer further illness if an ambulance did not arrive promptly. The claimant and the defendant were 'sufficiently proximate' once the London Ambulance Service accepted the call and dispatched an ambulance, and a specific duty of care was established. There was no good reason for it failing to arrive within a reasonable timeframe, so therefore this duty was breached. It was deemed to be 'fair, just and reasonable' to allow a duty of care to exist between an ambulance service and its patients, and such notions will be discussed in greater depth later in this chapter.

As a direct result of the Constitutional Reform Act 2005, the Supreme Court was set up to replace the House of Lords as the highest domestic court in England. The House of Lords was deemed to be a slightly confusing term for the final court of appeal, as it related both to the court and the upper chamber of Parliament that is occupied by peers as well as very senior judges. In 2009, the Supreme Court heard its first case, with the final case heard in the House of Lords being that of Debbie Purdy (*R (on the Application of Purdy) v Director of Public Prosecutions* (2009)), who was seeking clarification on the criminalisation of individuals who assist the terminally ill to commit suicide. The 'new' Supreme Court can hear appeals from the entire UK, a key factor in enabling the wider Union to be able to rely upon the judgement in the *Montgomery* case (*Montgomery v Lanarkshire Health Board* (2015)), as this originated in Scotland. The Court will always sit with an uneven number of judges to ensure that a case can be decided. This is typically five, though in the 2014 *Tony Nicklinson* case (*R (on the Application of Nicklinson and Another) v Ministry of Justice* (2014)), nine judges sat, with a 7:2 verdict being returned in favour of maintaining the current legal position on assisted suicide. Whilst this is holistically true, there were actually a number of questions before the Court, including those surrounding whether the current provision satisfies the specifics in Article 8 of the European Convention on Human Rights.

'In our view, therefore, medical law is a subset of human rights law' (Kennedy and Grubb 2000). The Human Rights Act 1998 forms the core of much of the body of applied law within medicine, and subjects allied to health. Negligence and breach of the duty of care tend to be the tortious activity, but the standards against which the acts are judged are most commonly drawn from the Human Rights Act.

Remedy

The outcomes of a successful (in terms of the person bringing the action) civil case will be one of a number of civil remedies which will be of benefit to the claimant. These remedies include damages in the form of compensation, and injunctions to compel the defendant to complete (or not complete) a specific action. The latter is less likely in cases brought against medical practitioners, as the relationship between the clinician and the patient is likely to have broken down at this time – even in cases where the paramedic may be practising within a non-acute setting such as aesthetics. The most likely outcome is damages being awarded against the individual paramedic or vicariously against the trust or organisation the paramedic is employed by.

The Criminal Courts

The path of a case through the criminal justice system is extremely different from that of a civil case. There is a requirement for more work to be undertaken in order to enable a case to get to court, and many cases fall prior to being heard in the magistrates' court. Criminal cases are brought by the state against individuals or companies (corporate defendants). The state includes the police as investigators, and the Crown Prosecution Service, which prepares the Crown's case against the defendant. There are numerous outcomes from a criminal trial and according to the Sentencing Council (2018), this 'can lead to the defendant(s) being convicted of an offence or offences either after a trial or because they plead guilty. Alternatively, they may be found not guilty, or the case may be halted before a conclusion is reached'. These outcomes depend upon whether the defendant pleads guilty or not guilty. If the defendant pleads guilty, they will then be committed for sentencing, which can be immediate or at a later date. The Sentencing Council (2018) notes that most cases end with a guilty plea even when they commence with a plea of not guilty. If the defendant pleads not guilty, they may be found guilty by the magistrate or a jury; again, they would be committed for a sentencing hearing as noted above. On occasion, a jury or magistrate may find the defendant not guilty of one offence but guilty of a lesser offence. This is permitted, but one cannot be found guilty of an unrelated offence at trial. If there is insufficient evidence to be confident of the offender's guilt, the case will end with a not guilty verdict or, in some instances, no verdict will be recorded. If the jury in a Crown Court case cannot reach a majority verdict, a hung jury will be called. As a result, the judge will dismiss the jury and the prosecution may ask for a re-trial; if this is not granted, the charges will be dropped and the case ends.

There are occasions when the trial concludes before a verdict is received. This may be because the prosecution does not have enough evidence to proceed and they may drop the case before it goes to trial. Alternatively, a judge or magistrate may throw out the case, for example, if key evidence is not available or if there is a reason why the defendant would not receive a fair trial. Whether the defendant can be tried at a later date for the same offence will depend on the circumstances of the individual case.

There are two distinct functions during the case-building phase. First, the police service is seen as the state's investigatory arm, and the Crown Prosecution Service will take this evidence and build a case if it fulfils a number of essential criteria. There needs to be a realistic prospect of securing a conviction from the evidence presented and the prosecution must be in the public interest. These guidelines are set out in the 2013 Code for Crown Prosecutors at paragraphs 4.7–4.12. The key questions centre on whether prosecution is an appropriate response, and in cases of negligence which touch the criminal sphere, this is often at the heart of the decision, as in the *Winterbourne View* case (*R v Rodgers and Others* (2012)). Second, the impact on the community is determined. This can be viewed as the paramedic profession, the local health system or the community from which the patient originates. Anecdotally, there seems to be reluctance to pursue criminal actions against the emergency services when a civil route is available and will provide a suitable recourse.

Unlike in civil cases, in criminal cases there are a wide range of sentences at the disposal of magistrates and judges. These can range from an absolute (where the defendant is found guilty and has a criminal record, but can walk free from court with no sanction other than the sentence) or conditional discharge, where certain conditions must be fulfilled. These conditions may include signing in at a police station on regular occasions or attending rehabilitation groups. At the other end of the spectrum is a life sentence, which would usually hold a tariff of a minimum time to be served before the defendant is able to apply for parole or release. A whole life sentence will ensure that the convicted defendant spends the rest of their life in prison.

A criminal case will enter the court system at the magistrates' court; at the initial hearing, it will be determined whether the case can be heard in the magistrates' court or if it will need to be transferred to the Crown Court. A magistrate sees summary offences and can sentence guilty parties to up to 6 months in prison, fine them up to £5,000 and impose community sentences such as unpaid community work. Indictable offences are presented in the Crown Court and will be heard in front of a judge and a jury, typically consisting of 12 lay persons or peers (though this is not to be confused with peers within the House of Lords). Triable either-way offences are offences that can be treated as either a summary offence or an indictable offence; thus, these offences are of mid-level seriousness, or whose seriousness may be the subject of debate.

The Court of Appeal and the Supreme Court

Once a case has been dealt with in the Crown Court, there are certain grounds under which it may be referred to the Criminal Division of the Court of Appeal – this includes if the conviction might be considered unsafe. This may be due to the evidence presented in the original trial, or new evidence that has been discovered since the date of the original trial. A decision from the Court of Appeal may also be granted leave of appeal to the Supreme Court. The Supreme Court often takes a more relaxed approach to binding precedents than in civil cases and looks more at the facts of each case being different, thus not overruling previous judgements, but rather distinguishing them on the basis of the facts.

Currently, there are no significantly documented cases of paramedics being at the heart of reported case law, as only those cases that reach the Court of Appeal or the Supreme Court are documented within the legal journals. That said, there is a body of evidence of how the criminal courts seek to protect paramedics and other emergency workers. In November 2006, the Emergency Workers (Obstruction) Act 2006 was introduced. In 2012, the government produced an evaluation of the law's effectiveness and, whilst it anticipated conviction rates to be low, the figures are rather stark. In the three years from 2007 to 2010, there were 26 cases commenced and, of those, 19 were found guilty and sentenced. The sentences received by those convicted of offences ranged from absolute discharge from duty to a fine and community sentence. Whilst there is no breakdown within the figures as to how many paramedic offences took place, this may demonstrate that the law, which can be used as a shield to protect emergency workers, might not be being utilised to its greatest extent. An overview of the court structure can be seen in Figure 4.2.

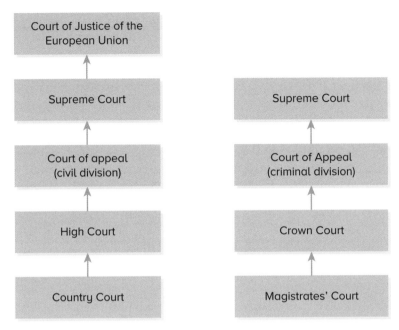

Figure 4.2 The passage hierarchy of the civil and criminal courts in England

When the Civil and Criminal Courts Collide

It has been emphasised that negligence is typically a matter for the civil courts, regardless of its degree. If gross negligence causes death, it may lead to a conviction of gross negligence manslaughter. This is a form of involuntary manslaughter, which is where the defendant was acting lawfully, but their actions, whilst lacking the necessary intent to satisfy murder, are criminally responsible for a person's death. This, unlike constructive manslaughter, can be committed by action or omission. The test for this was established in *R v Bateman* (1925) and affirmed in *Andrews v DPP* (1937). Failing to notice that a patient's endotracheal tube had become disconnected might render the paramedic liable for any negative consequences, as in the *Adomako* case (*R v Adomako* (1994)). However, a paramedic might in fact be protected due to the patient already being in cardiac arrest or by the fact that this is an emergency and the skill was performed in a life-or-death situation. The fact that Adomako failed to respond to the alarms is further evidence of his negligence. Following the *Adomako* case, it was necessary not only to satisfy the three basic needs to establish negligence – that a duty is owed, that there was a breach of the duty and that the duty resulted in a loss, in this case death – it was further noted that the defendant's conduct was so bad in all the circumstances as to amount to, in the jury's opinion, a crime. The threat of litigation for medical errors, however small, causes anxiety within a profession and threatens the advancement of the profession. Furthermore, it has been argued that clinicians should only face criminal proceedings if there is a blatant disregard for a patient's welfare, thus demonstrating some malice or intent in their actions.

It has been previously discussed that one of the longstanding principles that underpins the application of the criminal law to medical malpractice is that medics are normally only found to be criminally liable if the patient has died. A paramedic who is reckless with a patient's welfare and causes serious injury would likely face criminal proceedings. It has been a long-established provision that the wilful neglect of a mentally ill or mentally incapacitated patient under both the Mental Health Act 1983 and the Mental Capacity Act 2005 would be a crime, and this is now extended to patients with full decision-making capability. This was thought only to extend to doctors and nurses, but after the enactment of the Criminal Justice and Courts Act 2015 (sections 20–25), this has now been extended to all care providers, from care workers through to healthcare professionals such as paramedics. The focus of this Act is on the conduct of the individual rather than the outcome for the patient.

European Law and the European Courts

As a result of section 3(1) of the European Communities Act 1972, any decision of the Court of Justice of the European Union on issues relating to European law are binding upon all English courts. This said, the European court system sits outside of the English criminal justice system and the European Court of Justice only sits above the Supreme Court on matters concerning aspects of EU law. It is important to understand the distinction between the European Court of Justice and the European Court of Human Rights: the latter deals solely with alleged breaches of human rights by any Member State. The European Court of Justice typically deals with cases referred by the courts within each Member State or by the institutions of the EU, such as the European Commission, the European Parliament or the Council of Europe.

There are three main types of European legislation and their application is complex in comparison to the English legal system: these are treaties, regulations and directives. The impact on English law from these European provisions depends on a number of factors, such as direct applicability and direct effect. In essence, regulations are directly applicable and treaties are only directly applicable when domestic law is enacted. Therefore, each Member State is obliged to absorb these immediately into their legal systems. Directives are not directly applicable, but can have direct effect, though this has been challenged by many Member States. In order to rely directly upon a treaty, regulation or directive, it must be clear, unconditional and require no further legislation to enable an individual or a Member State to rely upon the provision. This test as laid out in *Van Gend en Loos v Nederlandse Tariefcommissie* (1963) has reinforced that this might be applicable to treaties and regulations, but this is rarely the case for directives.

Treaties

A European treaty effectively forms part of a European constitution. It has previously been discussed that the UK does not have written consultation apart from when it comes to the treaties of the EU. There are currently two functioning treaties: the Treaty on European Union (also known as the Maastricht Treaty) and the Treaty on the Functioning of the European Union (also known as the Rome Treaty). The treaties are not law in themselves and they still require domestic law to be enacted in order to enable their intentions to be applied in each Member State.

Regulations

Regulations are the closest piece of legislation that come out of Europe that reflects an English Act of Parliament. Regulations apply to Member States, but infer protection and provision for the general public and individuals, and do not typically need any specific law within each Member State as they become binding as soon as they are enacted. Regulations also have the power to trump existing domestic legislation and must be applied even if they are in direct conflict with passed legislation that is contradictory. This notion was tested in *Leonesio v Italian Ministry for Agriculture and Forestry* (1972), when the Italian government refused to adhere to the terms of a regulation to encourage reduced dairy function, stating that it required further legislation to make defect payments to farmers. The Italian ministry lost its case and was compelled to pay the farmer the money he was owed.

Directives

Directives are less precisely worded than regulations. They are usually set out as an overarching policy objective, leaving each Member State to develop their own legislation in order to put the directive in place within their domestic legal system. One directive familiar to ambulance service employees is the European Working Time Directive 93/104/EC, which restricted the number of hours staff could work in a day and also set out a minimum number of rest hours between shifts. This was later absorbed into English law as the *Working Time Directive 1998*. Directives can protect individuals from acts conducted by their government (vertical direct effect) and by private companies (horizontal direct effect). The influence of European law on practice is much more subtle than English domestic law, but there are cases that signal the intent of the EU to regulate activities of the state, which it is envisaged the ambulance service would fall under. The *Foster v British Gas* (1990) case broadened the concept of the state to include local authorities and other 'emanations of the state'. An emanation of the state can be described as '*a body, whatever its legal form, which has been made responsible, pursuant to a measure adopted by the state, for providing a public service under the control of the state and has for that purpose special powers beyond those which result from the normal rules applicable in relation between individuals* (1990, p. 20).

A further case which demonstrates the effectiveness of directives and how Member States are expected to set aside any current provisions which do not agree with EU law can be seen in *Marshall v Southampton and South West Hampshire Area Health Authority* (1986). Marshall challenged her employer's mandatory retirement age, which differed from that of her male counterparts, and requested that this issue was brought before the European Court of Justice by asking a question in accordance with Article 267 of the Treaty on European Union. The policy was legal under the relevant English legal provision, but was contrary to a European Council Directive. The European Court of Justice agreed that there was a conflict, and the UK was forced to change its legislation to reflect the EU provision.

With European legislation being more applicable to the state rather than the individual, and cases being referred to the Court of Justice being rather few and far between, the impact of European law on a day-to-day basis is not typically noticeable. The EU has been responsible for increased safety and equality within the workplace, but not for presiding over key cases that directly affect practice. That said, it would be wholly remiss for the European justice system to be ignored or set aside because of its limited day-to-day interaction within paramedic practice.

The full impact of the European Union (Notification of Withdrawal) Act 2017 has yet to be seen. Many European 'laws' are firmly ingrained within the English Legal system and there is currently no certainty that all this legislation will be rewound, repealed, set aside or watered down. Whilst there is a perception that the EU governed the colour of ambulances, this was only ever a voluntary EU Standard (CEN 1789:2007) rather than a rule that compelled the removal of white ambulances to be replaced with yellow ones, so it is likely these will remain yellow and green!

The Legal Framework of Decision Making

Decisions come with every patient interaction, some of which are clinical and others which are not. We may consider that we make these decisions in the best interests of our patients. However, how do we ensure that these are correct in the eyes of the law? The common law has built up a series of principles which establish good decision making. These have been tested through legal proceedings such as tribunals and ombudsman complaints to challenge what might be considered an unlawful decision. These principles note that the decision maker must identify the law correctly and ensure that they are aware of the boundaries of their legal power and that they do not extend this. This is extremely relevant in cases which relate to the Mental Capacity Act 2005 and mental capacity assessment. In supporting this, there is always an expectation that any statutory provision will be followed. The decision must be made in accordance with the purpose of the law; this is both the law as it is written and the spirit of the intention. This can be challenging, as it is not always clear what Parliament intended if it differs from the law as written. A further principle of good decision making is to take into account the requirements of natural justice, allowing all parties to have their say, avoiding any bias and reaching a decision based upon the weight of the evidence. It is also considered essential to act in good faith, thus avoiding discrimination and malice and applying the principles set out in the articles of the Human Rights Act 1998, which are relevant to all decisions of public bodies and their agents, of which a paramedic would be considered to fall within.

There are a number of circumstances where the misuse of power in the decision-making process has led to the decision maker being viewed by the courts to have acted unlawfully. On occasion, the law is applied incorrectly; this is known as illegality. The actions of the police officers in the *Sessay Case (R (Sessay) v South London and Maudsley NHS Foundation Trust* (2011)) may be considered to have acted in this way by utilising section 5 of the Mental Capacity Act 2005 to detain a patient rather than the police powers under section 136 of the Mental Health Act 1983. A second misuse of power would be improper purpose. This could be likened to a paramedic acting outside their scope of practice. It could be argued that being influenced by a patient's family or bystanders at the scene may lead to a decision being made without all the relevant considerations being taken into account; this could interfere with the ethical principle of justice. A decision may be considered unlawful if the outcome lacks proportionality; this is most commonly seen in mental capacity cases where a clinician is compelled to achieve the desired outcome through the least restrictive means possible (Mental Capacity Act 2005, Section 1(6)).

Legal Responsibility for Remote Advice

Remote and telephone advice has been an area of huge growth area in recent years not only within paramedic practice, but also within the wider NHS. Whilst this has been heralded as an ideal opportunity to 'take healthcare to the patient' or offer the 'right treatment at the right time in the right place', there is little formal clarification on the legal framework or position if something were to go wrong. Much of the professional guidance in this area comes from those agencies that represent professions that have been engaging in this activity for a number of years, such as the General Medical Council or the Nursing and Midwifery Council. For a clinician to be afforded such protection, a paramedic must act wholly within their scope of practice and follow procedures set out by their employers ensuring that their behaviour is congruent with both sets of practices. It is also key to be mindful that the same duty of care is held as would be the case in a face-to-face consultation. This is the key difference in terms of the assessment: a face-to-face assessment allows for the detection of visual cues, which is lost with telemedicine. Without legal precedent some confusion is likely to exist in this area as the National Institute for Health and Care Excellence (NICE), (2018) has called for further clarity to determine where the liability arises in remote clinical decision making.

Despite telephone consultations having inherent risks, it is how individual clinicians manage this risk which is key in ensuring litigation avoidance and the avoidance of negligence claims. There is also very little legislative support or control for telemedicine from a European perspective. Raposo (2016, p. 1–12) states that 'telemedicine is, simultaneously, a health service and an information service, therefore, both regulations apply. In what concerns healthcare and the practice of medicine there are no uniform regulations at the European level. Concerning health services, the most relevant achievement to regulate this domain is Directive 2011/24/EU. Regarding information and telecommunications, we must have in consideration Directive 95/46/EU, Directive 2000/31/EC and Directive 2002/58/EC, thus adding further confusion to the matter rather than creating any clarity. In addition, each directive Raposo discusses relates to criminality rather than tortious acts such as negligence or dereliction of a duty of care. It appears that remote advice will continue to be regulated by the standards and norms of traditional face-to-face consultations.

Contributory Negligence

The law surrounding contributory negligence remains unclear, as a number of cases which can easily be assimilated to ambulance work have all produced slightly conflicting outcomes and therefore varying legal precedents that could be relied upon. The Law Reform (Contributory Negligence) Act 1945 sets out that if a person is injured partly as a result of their own actions despite some negligent act being noted, they would be subject to reduced damages, as in the case of *Horsley v Cascade Insulation Services and Others* (2009). Trevor Horsley was not injured by negligent medical treatment, but developed asbestosis from years of working in a factory. In addition, he was also a heavy smoker and, despite having received smoking cessation advice on numerous occasions, continued to smoke. He was found to have contributed to his respiratory disability and therefore his ability to claim damages was diminished. In comparison, in *St George v Home Office* (2008), an alcohol-dependent patient who was suffering from withdrawal was assigned a top bunk in the hospital. The patient had a withdrawal seizure and as a consequence suffered a brain injury and was left with long-term brain damage. The courts found that, despite the patient's withdrawing state and subsequent seizure being a consequence of an unwise or reckless act, this did not constitute negligence in the eyes of the law and therefore the hospital was solely responsible for the loss as it had negligently placed the patient in the top bunk. This is akin to securing your patient on the stretcher; the fact that they may be intoxicated or under the influence of any other substance would unlikely be a defence to any negligence claims brought against the ambulance crew.

Private Practice

With the steady evolution of the scope of paramedic practice and the distinct movement away from traditional NHS ambulance services, there has been a significant growth in paramedics entering the private sector. With that comes a different set of responsibilities over and above what has already been discussed earlier in this chapter. A patient who pays for treatment or a provision of care enters into a contract with the paramedic. The paramedic is free to set the terms of the contract, except that they cannot exempt themselves from liability for any injury or adverse outcome that may arise from a negligent act, as this would be contrary to section 2 of the Unfair Contract Terms Act 1977 and also extremely ethically questionable. In private practice, a paramedic may be held in breach of contract for failing to deliver a promised outcome, though this is likely to be through contracted services rather than patient outcomes. This would never happen within the NHS as the paramedic would only be liable for a tortious act, such as negligence.

Summary

Specific laws relating to the paramedic are rather sparse, but there are many key principles that can be inferred onto paramedic practice. The civil courts generate much of the case law that governs how paramedics act, and what the expectations of the courts and public are towards a regulated profession. With the significant expansion of the paramedic role, it might be expected that we will see further challenges within the courts in the years to come, in much the same way as we have seen a steady increase in litigation involving the medical professions. When paramedicine starts to move within the fields traditionally governed by general practice, there may well be an increase in ambulance-related litigation. However, until then, the legal framework to operate as a paramedic remains within the solid basis of law, which provides guidance on the expectation of the modern paramedic.

Recommended Reading

Brazier, M and Cave, E (2017) *Medicine, Patients and the Law*, 6th ed. Manchester: Manchester University Press.

Elliott, C and Quinn, F (2017) *English Legal System*, 18th ed. Harlow: Pearson.

Slapper, G and Kelly, D (2015) *The English Legal System*, 16th ed. London: Routledge.

Bogdanor, V (2001) *Devolution in the UK*. Oxford: Oxford University Press.

References

Bennion FAR (2005) *Statutory Interpretation*. London: Butterworths.

Blackstone, W (1765) *Commentaries on the Laws of England Vol 1*. Oxford: Clarendon Press.

Dicey, A (1982) *Introduction to the Study of Law of the Constitution*. Indianapolis: Library Classics.

Kennedy, I and Grubb, A (2000) *Medical Law*, 3rd ed. London: Butterworths.

National Institute for Health and Care Excellence (2018) Chapter 4 Paramedic Remote Support. *Emergency and acute medical care in over 16s: service delivery and organisation*. Available at www.nice.org.uk/guidance/ng94/evidence/04.paramedic-remote-support-pdf-4788818465.

Raposo, VL (2016) Telemedicine: the legal framework (or the lack of it) in Europe. *GMS Health Technology Assessment*, 12. Available at: www.ncbi.nlm.nih.gov/pmc/articles/PMC4987488/pdf/HTA-12-03.pdf.

Sentencing Council (2018) *Criminal trial outcomes*. Available at: www.sentencingcouncil.org.uk/about-sentencing/information-for-victims/trial-outcomes.

UK Cases

A Practice Direction [1991] 3 All ER 722

Andrews v DPP [1937] AC 576

Beard v London General Omnibus Company [1900] 2 QB 530

Bolam v Friern Hospital Management Committee [1957] 1 WLR 582

Cusack v London Borough of Harrow [2013] UKSC 40

Horsley v Cascade Insulation Services and Others [2009] EWHC 2945

Kent v Griffiths [2000] 2 All ER 474

Limpus v London General Omnibus Company [1861] 158 ER 993

Montgomery v Lanarkshire Health Board [2015] SC 11; [2015] 1 AC 1430

R v Adomako [1994] 4 All ER 935

R v Bateman [1925] 19 Cr App R 8

R (on the Application of Nicklinson and Another) v Ministry of Justice; R (on the Application of AM) v Director of Public Prosecutions [2014] UKSC 38

R (on the Application of Purdy) v Director of Public Prosecutions [2009] UKHL 45

R v Rodgers and Others [2012] unreported

R (Sessay) v South London and Maudsley NHS Foundation Trust [2011] EWHC 2617

Sidaway v Board of Governors of the Bethlem Royal Hospital and Others [1985] 871 AC

St George v Home Office [2008] EWCA Civ 1068

EU Cases

Foster and others v British Gas plc ECJ [1991] 2 WLR 258, [1990] 2 CMLR 833, 2 CMLR 833 ECJ, C-188/89, [1990] ECR I-3313,

Leonesio v Italian Ministry for Agriculture and Forestry [1972] ECR 287

Marshall v Southampton and South West Hampshire Area Health Authority [1986] ECR 723

Van Gend en Loos v Nederlandse Tariefcommissie (26/62) [1963] ECR 8 90 91

UK Legislation

Civil Procedure Act 1997

Civil Procedure Rules 1998

Constitutional Reform Act 2005

Criminal Justice and Courts Act 2015

European Communities Act 1972

European Union (Notification of Withdrawal) Act 2017

Government of Wales Act 1998

Human Rights Act 1998

Law Reform (Contributory Negligence) Act 1945

Mental Capacity Act 2005

Mental Health Act 1983

Northern Ireland Act 1998

Scotland Act 1998

Unfair Contract Terms Act 1977

Working Time Directive 1998

EU Legislation

Treaty on European Union

Directive 95/46/EU

Directive 93/104/EC

Directive 2000/31/EC

Directive 2002/58/EC

Directive 2011/24/EU

Chapter 5

Information Governance: Data Protection and Confidentiality

Keiran Bellis

Introduction

Information governance is the relationship between how we collect, hold, store, manage and use information in line with legal, moral and ethical codes within the principles of best practice. This underpins every patient interaction, from an initial meeting to completing all relevant documentation and providing a clinician-to-clinician handover. Information governance can impact upon the tripartite relationship between the patient, the employee and the employer in many ways. From a patient perspective, any breach of information governance will not only affect them personally, but may also impact upon their confidence in their care and their confidence in the service or the NHS as a whole. The employee and the clinician will also be affected. Any breaches may affect the employee's personal and professional reputation, and impact upon their registration if they are a registered professional. Finally, the employer, whether an ambulance service, wider NHS trust or private organisation, faces a loss of reputation alongside the significant financial penalties which accompany breaches as well as costs in terms of redress, compensation and settlements.

This chapter will outline the legal and ethical mechanisms that underpin confidentiality, data protection and information governance in relation to paramedic practice.

Data Protection

A core element of information governance is data protection. This is the legal term coined to ensure that there are safe systems for the collection, storage and destruction of personal data. As a consequence of patient interactions, data is naturally generated, with some being highly personal. Therefore, strong legislative frameworks and safe systems are extremely pertinent in all aspects of healthcare. The legal landscape supporting data protection was developing long before the original Data Protection Act 1998, with much of the policy being shaped by the EU in Brussels. Data protection within the UK has not been subject to devolved legislation, which means that all nations are bound by the same laws. That said, a strong legislative framework has only been seen in the UK since the 1984 and 1998 Acts.

Reviewing the foundations of data protection laws, some of the earliest mentions of this new phenomenon were made by two American lawyers, Samuel D. Warren and Louis Brandeis, in 1890. Warren and Brandeis wrote a paper entitled 'The right to privacy', which argued that every person deserves the right 'to be left alone'. This has subsequently been used as a definition of privacy, which is reflected in much of the subsequent legislation. Despite this shaping the language of the future, there was little formal or legal advancement for many years until the adoption of the 1948 Universal Declaration of Human Rights, which held privacy as the twelfth fundamental right. This is now Article 8 of the Human Rights Act 1998. In 1950, the EU Convention on Human Rights amended the sequence, but this acted as a timely reinforcement of the 'new' rights and the protection the Convention afforded to the individual against other individuals, industry and other EU Member States. This maintained a period of legislative stability for many years until 1981, when the EU's Council of Europe adopted the Data Protection Convention (Treaty 108), which now described the right to privacy as 'a legal imperative' rather than a broadly accepted right. The UK first enacted the Data Protection Act 1984, which set out key principles according to which data collection was to be conducted and how that data was held. This piece of legislation was short lived as it was repealed in 1998 by the Data Protection Act 1998, which enacted the 1995 European Data Protection Directive (Directive 95/46/EC). At the time, this piece of legislation was the single largest development in data protection legislation and saw a renewed focus upon the way in which data was handled at each stage of its management. A series of new terms such as data processing, sensitive data and consent were also introduced. It is the notion of consent which underpins many of the interactions paramedics face during daily clinical care. With the development of technology and specifically digital technology, it was considered that the current legal framework, both within the UK and the wider EU, was no longer fit for purpose.

> The Council of Europe is an arm of the EU whose aims are to uphold key rights such as the rule of law, democracy and human rights.

The world has changed significantly in the 20 years since the 1998 Act was passed. New technology and social networks make it easier than ever to access, use and share data. This is why it is important to ensure data protection laws are fit for the age we live in. There were a number of years of legislative turmoil where numerous breaches and leaks of patient data were uncovered, and it was identified that more could and should be done to protect individuals against such events. Legislation from the EU was passed down, enacted (Directive 2006/24/EC, Directive 2002/58/EC and Regulation 2013/611) and declared invalid by the Court of Justice for violation of other fundamental rights (Directive 2006/24/EC). However, this type of piecemeal legal framework often leads to uncertainty in both the courts and in the day-to-day activity of patient data collection, management and storage. Finally, in 2018, after over four years of discussions, the European General Data Protection Regulation (Regulation 2016/679) was approved by the EU and enacted within UK legislation in 2018. The law by which it has been embedded in UK legislation is now known as the Data Protection Act 2018. The 2018 Act, through the General Data Protection Regulation (GDPR), brings everyone up to date by strengthening and unifying data protection for all individuals within the EU.

The Data Protection Act 2018

What Does the Act Do?

The 2018 Act makes data protection laws for the modern digital age and its content reflects the vast amount of data which is being processed on a daily basis. This also empowers individuals to take control of who sees, uses and stores their data, whilst ensuring that the nation's data protection systems are fit for purpose after the UK leaves the EU.

What are the Key Elements of the Act?

- *General data protection*
  - Implements the EU General Data Protection Regulation.
  - Ensures that sensitive health, social care and education data can continue to be processed, whilst making sure that confidentiality in health and safeguarding situations are maintained.
  - Provides appropriate restrictions to rights of access and to delete data held, affirming the right to be forgotten.
  - Sets the age from which parental consent is not needed to process data online at 13 years old. However, this is not a blanket age limit across all data protection and disclosure environments, as healthcare-specific cases will keep their current thresholds.
- *Law enforcement*
- *Intelligence services processing*
- *Regulation and enforcement*
  - Gives greater power to the Information Commissioner to regulate and enforce data protection rules.
  - Increases the fines to data controllers and processors, including public and private bodies. This will include ambulance services and the wider NHS.
  - Empowers the Information Commissioner to consider and bring criminal proceedings against offences where the Data Controller is intent on preventing a lawful disclosure.

How Will This Affect Paramedics?

- In general terms, it has not had a noticeable impact as patient care has been unaffected.
- It has likely had an impact on the health promotion and research function of pre-hospital medicine.
- Any breach impacts the NHS Trust, private company and health service financially and vicariously due to the increased fine levy.

Confidentiality

I will respect the secrets which are confided in me, even after the patient has died.

Declaration of Geneva (as amended in 2016)

A key notion within paramedic practice and naturally the wider healthcare systems is that of confidentiality and the duty of paramedics to maintain confidentiality. This duty arises from a number of sources – from the legislation discussed above and the individual's professional codes as well as their contract of employment.

The notion of confidentiality is significantly more established than that of data protection, yet this has greater direct relevance to the day-to-day activity of healthcare at the 'sharp end' than to traditional data protection activity. All practitioners within healthcare must demonstrate the ability to both maintain confidence and a knowledge of the process of when to share relevant information with other agencies. In order for medical care to be effective, there must be trust between the patient and the clinician. That trust is built on many things, including competence, empathy and confidence that the clinician will keep the consultation confidential.

The Health and Care Professions Council (HCPC) (2016) defines confidentiality as 'protecting personal information. This information might include details of a service user's lifestyle, family, health or care needs which they want to be kept private'. The rules and legal frameworks supporting confidentiality, and more specifically disclosure, have been built up in a rather piecemeal manner. Despite all the varying codes of conduct, ethical codes and supporting legislation, there is no single piece of guidance which affirms a clinician's duty in relation to data protection, confidentiality and disclosure.

The law supporting breach of confidence has again developed in a very piecemeal fashion. As noted above, there is no single law supporting this, so clinicians must factor in duties from a number of differing sources. The overarching basis upon which a medical duty of confidentiality as set out by Boreham J in *Hunter v Mann* (1974) is that: 'The doctor is under a duty not to disclose, without consent of his patient, information which he, the doctor, has gained in his professional capacity save . . . in very exceptional circumstances.'

Hunter v Mann (1974)

A doctor who failed to disclose information linking the patient to a hit-and-run accident was convicted and fined under section 168(2) of the Road Traffic Act 1972. The doctor was under a duty to inform the police of his patient's involvement in the incident. Discretionary disclosure is subject to the public interest exception.

When considering the law which governs patient confidentiality, it is imperative that the Human Rights Act 1998 is considered, with special attention to both Article 8 (right to privacy), and to a lesser extent Article 10 (freedom of expression). Article 8(1) of the Human Rights Act 1998 states that: 'Everyone has the right to respect for his private and family life, his home and his correspondence.' In supporting this, the European Court of Human Rights has constantly upheld this right in relation to the disclosure and access to patients' medical records. The information which is disclosed during the course of patient assessment and treatment form this record. That said, it must be further considered that this is a qualified right and not an absolute right such as the right to life (Article 2), so, as with the judgement laid down in *Hunter v Mann*, there will be times this duty can be circumvented. This might be in the course of a criminal investigation (*Z v Finland* (1997)) or in the assessment of social security or state benefits (*MS v Sweden* (1997)). The Human Rights Act further notes (in Article 8(2)) that 'in accordance with the law and as necessary in democratic society, in the interests of national security public safety, or the economic well-being of the country, for the prevention of disorder or a crime, for the protection of health or morals, or for the protection of the rights and freedoms of others' it may at times be appropriate to disclose information for the safety of others. The specific duty of the paramedic will be discussed later on in this chapter, and the ethics concerning this (utilitarianism) were discussed in Chapter 3.

A key case in the evolution of confidentiality protection comes not from the medical arena, but from the media. In *Campbell v Mirror Group Newspapers* (2002), the principle of the duty of confidence and confidentiality was tested in the highest court of the land (at the time this was the House of Lords; as noted previously, this is now the Supreme Court). In the case, there was a significant discussion of what should and could be considered confidential, and whether the term 'private' was more palatable. This is extremely pertinent within the healthcare field as promises of confidentiality cannot always necessarily be upheld, and there is a duty to share certain pieces of information with other agencies in relation to both protecting the patient and others. Lord Nicholls stated in the *Campbell* case that: 'The continuing use of the phrase "duty of confidence" and the description of the information as "confidential" is not altogether comfortable. Information about an individual's private life would not, in ordinary usage, be called "confidential". The more natural description today is that such information is private. The essence of the tort is better encapsulated now as misuse of private information.' This terminology has been confirmed and adopted in a number of subsequent cases, such as *Hutchinson (formerly KGM) v News Group Newspapers Ltd* (2011) and *Viddal-Hall v Google Inc.* (2015). These do not relate specifically to medical cases, but do provide quite specific principles on what should be followed within subsequent cases.

Caldicott Principles

Combining the fact that much of the reported case law regarding this sits outside of the medical sphere and the increasing worries concerning the use of patient information in the NHS, the need to avoid the undermining of confidentiality in the light of expanding technology is crucial. A review was therefore commissioned in 1997 by the Chief Medical Officer of England. This was the Caldicott Review, and the Caldicott Committee's Report on the Review of Patient-Identifiable Information (usually referred to as the Caldicott Report) was first published in 1997, which introduced six principles for data protection and confidentiality within health and social care. Despite being published over 20 years ago, these principles are still the cornerstone for the management of patient data and the revised (2013) principles are outlined below.

Principle 1: Justify the Purpose(s) for Using Confidential Information

The first principle highlighted by Dame Fiona Caldicott was the requirement to justify the purpose for using confidential information. In essence, each proposed use or transfer of personal confidential data within or from an organisation should be clearly defined, scrutinised and documented, with continuing uses regularly reviewed, by an appropriate guardian. It was foreseen that this would be the organisation's Caldicott guardian, a specific named individual who would act as a single point of contact for confidentiality and data protection advice and guidance. Such guidance might be sought from a staff member by a patient or member of the public.

Principle 2: Don't Use Personal Confidential Data Unless it is Absolutely Necessary

The second principle states that personal confidential data should not be used unless it is absolutely necessary. Personal confidential data items should not be included unless these are essential for the specified purpose. The need for patients to be identified should be considered at each stage of satisfying the purpose.

Principle 3: Use the Minimum Necessary Personal Confidential Data

The third principle requires the minimum necessary personal confidential data to be sought to achieve the desired outcome. Where use of personal confidential data is considered to be essential, the inclusion of each individual item of data should be considered, and justified, so that the minimum amount of personal confidential data is transferred or accessible as is necessary for a given function to be carried out.

Principle 4: Access to Personal Confidential Data Should Be on a Strict Need-to-Know Basis

The fourth principle is key within pre-hospital care, given how many clinician-to-clinician handovers often take place in public departments or over the phone. This indicated that access to personal confidential data should be on a strict need-to-know basis. Only those individuals who need access to personal confidential data should have access to it, and they should only have access to the data items that they need to see. This may mean controlling who has sight of personal records and information.

Principle 5: Everyone with Access to Personal Confidential Data Should Be Aware of Their Responsibilities

The fifth principle states that everyone with access to personal confidential data should be aware of their responsibilities. Action should be taken to ensure that those handling personal confidential data have the correct governance to do so. This extends to both clinical and non-clinical staff, and these staff members must be made fully aware of their responsibilities and obligations to respect patient confidentiality.

Principle 6: Comply with the Law

It is expected that all who collect and manage patient data will comply with the law. This means that every use of personal confidential data should be lawful. Someone in each organisation handling personal confidential data should be responsible for ensuring that the organisation complies with legal requirements and that as a result of the expectations of the fifth principle, each individual will be aware of their own legal requirements.

Principle 7: The Duty to Share Information Can Be as Important as the Duty to Protect Patient Confidentiality

In April 2013, Dame Fiona Caldicott reported on her second review of information governance. Her report, 'Information: To Share or Not to Share? The Information Governance Review', informally known as the Caldicott 2 Review, introduced a new final (seventh) principle. This new principle states that the duty to share information can be as important as the duty to protect patient confidentiality. Health and social care professionals should have the confidence to share information in the best interests of their patients within the framework set out by these principles. They should be supported by the policies of their employers, regulators and professional bodies. This disclosure is key and has been a key element of data protection and confidentiality within health and social care for a number of years.

Disclosures

The disclosure of private (or confidential) patient information may be permitted in a limited number of cases. These are set out below and have been subject to significant scrutiny over recent years. These disclosures will fall into one of two key categories: statutory or voluntary disclosures. Just because they are voluntary does not mean that there is no legal basis for the disclosure, but rather that the disclosure is not based on an Act of Parliament. Despite this, not all disclosures are made without consent. As we have previously established, paramedics along with all other healthcare professionals hold a duty of care to keep patients' personal information confidential (*Furniss v Fitchett* (1958)). Accompanying this is the right of any patient who satisfies a mental capacity assessment to waive this right and give consent for their information to be shared. An example of this can be seen in clinician-to-clinician handovers in emergency departments and urgent care centres across the length and breadth of the country, often with consideration to how a patient's personal information is being managed. This consent must be freely obtained before the transfer of information occurs and this can be sought in written or oral form.

Statutory Disclosure

There is on occasion a legal requirement to disclose health information, regardless of whether consent has been obtained for the disclosure, but there are strict guidelines in order for such a disclosure to be lawful. One common disclosure arises from a public health perspective and most notably serious communicable diseases. Section 11 of the Public Health (Control of Disease) Act 1984 requires that those involved within healthcare must notify the 'proper authorities' about certain infectious diseases. There is also an additional duty on physicians registered with the General Medical Council (GMC) (2009) to consider alerting the relevant individuals as to other infectious diseases such as HIV and AIDS. This remains extremely controversial and there is currently no explicit duty set out by the HCPC. The AIDS (Control) Act 1987 states that the disease is not notifiable and thus limits the duty of physicians in terms of making disease specific disclosures.

There are a number of provisions within the Children Act 1989 which are relevant to information sharing and specifically to the legal power to disclose personal information. Section 27 of the Act requires other agencies to help social care carry out its duties under section 17, as long as to do so is compatible with their own statutory duties and that by doing so they would not unduly prejudice the discharge of their own functions.

A defence to making a disclosure without consent would be in order to assist in the prevention or detection of a serious crime. It is important to remember that the police and lawyers do not have any automatic powers to demand disclosure or to demand any form of medical information, and they must apply for a court order to obtain this, unless the information is used in the prevention or detection of a serious crime. That said, medics are rarely experts in terms of what amounts to a serious crime and a judge can find a clinician to be in contempt of court for failing to provide the relevant information to assist in the detection of the aforementioned serious offence. The Criminal Law Act 1967 and the Police and Criminal Evidence Act 1984 (PACE) offer some guidance as to what might be considered such an offence, with PACE stating that a serious offence is one giving rise to a risk to national security, interfering with justice and causing death or serious injury. It is also under the auspices of this Act that the police would obtain powers to access medical records. In addition, disclosure also arises from the general global duty contained in section 19 of the Terrorism Act 2000 to inform the police if an individual believes or suspects terrorist-related activity. This is further reinforced by an additional duty in the Terrorism Act 2006 and the Prevention of Terrorism Act 2005. As noted earlier, in the judgement in the *Hunter v Mann* (1974) case, the Road Traffic Act 1991 requires medical practitioners to give patient details to the police when the driver is alleged to have committed an offence under the Act, and a failure to do so may result in prosecution.

Voluntary Disclosure

At the heart of voluntary disclosure is often the notion of the public interest. This may be to prevent harm to the public at large or a specific group within society. Much of the discussion regarding public interest disclosure centres on what is in the public interest and what the public may be interested in. There is a defence towards the former, but certainly not the latter. There are two significant cases at the heart of whether a public interest disclosure can be considered lawful. In *X v Y* (1998), information pertaining to the AIDS status of two doctors was obtained by a breach of confidence by a member of the Health Authority's staff. Upon reflection and in summarising, Rose J stated that in reviewing the likelihood of physician-to-patient infection and that the necessary counselling about safe practice had taken place, there were no public interests arguments which outweighed the requirement to maintain confidence.

X v Y (1998)

A Health Authority sought an injunction to prevent a national newspaper publishing the names of two practising doctors who were receiving treatment for AIDS. The court balanced the public interest in freedom of the press against the public interest in keeping hospital records confidential. It found that a lack of publication of the information would be of minimal significance, since there was a wide-ranging public debate about AIDS generally.

In balancing these competing interests, it should be noted that disclosure should in any event only be made to a relevant party. As a result, there should be no blanket disclosure.

This is contrasted with the case of *W v Edgell* (1989), where the Court of Appeal sanctioned a breach in a patient's confidence to ensure public safety. It must be noted that the Court of Appeal made it clear that Dr Edgell did hold a duty of confidence on all other aspects of his care and it was solely the fact that W (the patient) remained a danger to the wider public upon their release into the community. If Dr Edgell had written graphically regarding W's care in his memoirs or had sold his story to the press, he would have been in breach of W's confidence.

W v Edgell (1989)

The doctor–patient relationship is one in which information divulged by patients imposes a duty of confidence. In *W v Edgell*, the claimant, a convicted murderer, applied for a transfer to a less secure hospital as a step towards his release into a community hospital. His lawyers sought an independent psychiatric report from Dr Edgell, who concluded that the patient (W) was still a danger to the public. His advisers then withdrew the application. However, Dr Edgell chose to send the report to the medical director of the secure hospital and the Home Office. When W discovered this, he sought an injunction restraining disclosure of the report and damages for breach of confidence. The court found for the defendant, Dr Edgell, as the breach was justified in the public interest. W appealed and lost. The Court of Appeal accepted that the obligation of confidence was not absolute, especially where there was a stronger public interest in disclosure. Where this is the case, disclosure can only be justified when it is necessary to counter a specific threat and, thus, a foreseeable danger of serious or physical harm. In such a situation, the doctor would have a duty of care to the potential victim.

> **Pause for Thought**
>
> *Do paramedics and pre-hospital practitioners have a duty to report that a patient has suffered from a seizure or seizure-related activity to a receiving doctor, given the increased duty that a doctor may be under to report this to the Driver Vehicle Licensing Agency (DVLA), especially if this seizure is unwitnessed?*

According to Brazier and Cave (2017), the paramedic faces an ethical balancing act in terms of weighing up the harm done to the patient (and the public trust) by breaching confidence against the patient should an adverse event occur, with the risks potentially being very low. The GMC published guidance in 2009 (GMC 2009) which advises doctors that in such a case, they not only may but should contact the DVLA. As a consequence, it might be considered that paramedics shoulder a degree of the burden to inform the receiving hospital of their concerns.

Disclosure When the Patient Lacks Capacity

Under the Mental Capacity Act 2005, there is a presumption of capacity. In the case of patients with sufficient capacity, permission for any disclosure should be sought unless the patient cannot clearly articulate what has been discussed. In patients who lack capacity, there remains a key question of how much information should be shared with others who might have an interest in the patient's care. Section 4(7) of the Mental Capacity Act 2005 indicates that there is a duty, wherever practicable, to consult with the appropriate persons about their treatment. Discussing the treatment option of an unconscious patient with colleagues and the patient's family would be deemed an appropriate, proper and lawful option (*R (on the Application of S) v Plymouth City Council* (2002)). However, when the patient is alert and refusing to consent to the disclosure, the clinician will need to be certain that the patient lacks capacity to lawfully share information with others. Further, only information which is essential to share should be disclosed at this time, and in general there is no need to discuss previous injuries or medical treatments. An example would be if a patient is unconscious after suffering serious head and abdominal injuries. It may be lawful for the clinicians to discuss the patient's current condition and prognosis, but not to disclose that examinations show that they have had previous unrelated surgery.

Disclosure to Protect the Patient

The most common reason for paramedics making a disclosure in order to protect a patient would be to safeguard vulnerable patients. Professional guidance within the *Standards of Proficiency – Paramedics* (HCPC 2014) suggests that paramedics should be able to understand the importance of being able to maintain confidentiality, whilst being able to recognise and respond appropriately to situations where it is necessary to share information to safeguard service users or the wider public.

It seems that death also affects the obligation to maintain patient confidentiality. Since the case of *Lewis v Secretary of State for Health* (2008), it has been established that the duty to maintain confidence is capable of surviving a patient's death and Foskett J noted that this was key in maintaining public expectations of the health service and the profession. What was unclear was the length of time for which this duty existed, as the legal obligation was not considered to be permanent and the period of time may depend on the sensitivity of the information and any surviving relatives who may be harmed by the disclosure.

Remedies for Breach of Confidence

As breach of confidence is a civil tort rather than a criminal offence, there are a number of remedies at the court's disposal. One such remedy would be an injunction. A patient can apply to the court for an injunction to restrain publication of confidential information in full or in part. The court has discretionary power to do this. If this is not appropriate, the court may seek a declaration, which is where the claimant may be satisfied with a declaration from the court that an anticipated disclosure will amount to a breach of confidence or that a breach has actually taken place.

Punitive damages may be paid where a breach of confidence has caused financial harm to the patient by affecting the patient's business opportunities or employment prospects; such losses could be compensated. Where the harm is cited as anxiety or mental stress, the law is less certain about what, if any, damages can be recovered. However, in *Lady Archer v Williams* (2003), the claimant received £2,500 in damages for breach of confidence and injury to feelings. Restitutionary damages may be payable where those responsible for the breach make financial gain by breaching a confidence – for example, by selling a patient's story to the press, it is likely that the patient will be awarded the earned profits. This is seen more in celebrity doctors' memoirs rather than the published diary of a paramedic.

The Controlled Sharing of Information

Two further pieces of legislation exist to provide a lawful framework for the sharing of patient data, though they have been developed for differing reasons: first, the National Health Service Act 2006 (specifically section 251); and, second, the provisions set out in the Health and Social Care Act 2012, which created the Health and Social Care Information Centre (HSCIC). These pieces of legislation will support health promotion and research, which are two significant growth areas within paramedic practice. Like the GDPR and the Data Protection Act 2018, these may not have a direct relevance to the core function of the ambulance service, but awareness of such legislation is important.

The NHS Act 2016

Section 251 of the NHS Act 2006 (formerly section 60 of the Health and Social Care Act 2001) provides a statutory power to allow the Secretary of State for Health to set aside the need to obtain informed consent to ensure that NHS patient-identifiable information (which is needed to support essential NHS activity) can be used without the consent of patients. This is unlikely to affect paramedics on a daily basis, but could extend to the collection of datasets during the patient assessment process. This power can only be used to support medical purposes which are in the best interests of the wider public where consent is not practicable or where anonymised data will not suffice. Currently, this applies only to England and Wales, with similar arrangements across the rest of the UK though their devolved powers. In Scotland, patient information is brought together and managed at a national level by the Information Services Division of NHS Scotland. This does not have the power to disclose identifiable information without consent; the only option to make mass disclosures in Scotland is to rely upon a public interest disclosure. Northern Ireland's Privacy Advisory Committee can advise on many of the considerations as described in the section 251 provision, but it lacks statutory powers. Although section 251 can temporarily set aside the common law duty of confidentiality, compliance with all other aspects of the Data Protection Act 2018 must still be adhered to and the data must be collected, maintained and used in accordance with the Act.

The Health and Social Care Act 2012

The creation of the HSCIC as a result of the Health and Social Care Act 2012 has led to specific arrangements for data sharing in the non-acute context. The HSCIC is England's central repository of health and social care information for secondary and research purposes. It can require care providers to send certain datasets, including those containing confidential data, as a statutory requirement under section 256 of the Health and Social Care Act. The HSCIC will then publish this data for the wider use within healthcare research. However, this is not a carte blanche green light to share confidential information, as confidential information can only be released where there is a legal and ethical basis to do so (which will be discussed in Chapter 15). If there is no legal basis, the data can be produced to reflect this, which eradicates the risk to the research teams of datasets becoming compromised. The Health and Social Care Information Centre (2014) has issued a code of conduct concerning the request, management and use of confidential information. The principles within this code are also seen to have addressed some of the concerns which remained following the implementation of the Care Act 2012, namely the omission of the requirement to consult with patients where a disclosure is not designed to benefit them directly.

Patients' Access to Medical Records

As much as there is a requirement to protect the confidentiality of the patient, consideration must also be given to allowing a patient access to see the records which are held about them. There are various legislative procedures which permit access to a patient's own medical records and to those of deceased relatives. The first piece of legislation that offered individuals access to their medical records was the Access to Health Records Act 1990, which, despite containing many elements repealed by later Acts, is still on the statute books when considering deceased patients. This allows family members, and the executors of the deceased's estate, to view medical records held about the deceased. The overarching problem with the 1990 Act was that only the new, rather than historical, records were viewed. An attempt to create a common law right of access to all health records failed in 1995, with a challenge brought in the case of *R v Mid-Glamorgan Family Health Services ex parte Martin* (1995). As a consequence of this failure, the statutory picture remained confusing until 1998, when a general duty of access was established though the Data Protection Act 1998. This afforded patients a right of access to their full medical record. However, this duty only apples to living subjects. The Data Protection Act 2018 has further strengthened patients' access to their own medical records and general data which is held about them. It has harmonised conditions for the collection and use of health data by reducing timeframes and cost, allowing safe and appropriate access to data by the individual, clinicians and researchers alike.

Summary

Information governance encompasses data collection and patient confidentiality. The law regarding the use of patient information has been strengthened significantly since the enactment of the Data Protection Act 2018 following the EU's GDPR. This piece of legislation has drawn together much of the piecemeal legislation within this field, ensuring data protection and confidentiality in terms of how data is obtained, stored, managed and disposed of. Despite this, there is still a heavy reliance upon the common law system to support disclosure, specifically that without statutory underpinnings. The paramedic needs to be aware of the importance of information governance, regardless of their pillar of practice, setting of employment, or place of work.

Recommended Reading

Brazier, M and Cave, E (2017) *Medicine, Patients and the Law*, 6th ed. Manchester: Manchester University Press.

Carey, P (ed) (2018) *Data Protection: A Practical Guide to UK and EU Law*, 5th ed. Oxford: Oxford University Press.

Dimond, B (2010) *Legal Aspects of Patient Confidentiality*, 2nd ed. Huntingdon: Quay Publishing.

McHale, JV (1993) *Medical Confidentiality and Legal Privilege*. London: Routledge

Patteneden, R (2003) *The Law of Professional–Client Confidentiality: Regulating the Disclosure of Confidential Information*. Oxford: Oxford University Press.

References

Brazier, M and Cave, E (2017) *Medicine, Patients and the Law*, 6th ed. Manchester: Manchester University Press.

Council of Europe (1950) *European Convention for the Protection of Human Rights and Fundamental Freedoms, as amended by Protocols Nos. 11 and 14*. Available at: www.echr.coe.int/Documents/Convention_ENG.pdf.

Department of Health (1997) *Caldicott Committee Report on the Review of Patient-Identifiable Information*. Available at: http://static.ukcgc.uk/docs/caldicott1.pdf.

General Medical Council (GMC) (2009) *Confidentiality: disclosing information about serious communicable diseases*. Available at: www.gmc-uk.org/ethical-guidance/ethical-guidance-for-doctors/confidentiality—disclosing-information-about-serious-communicable-diseases.

Health and Care Professions Council (HCPC) (2014) *Standards of Proficiency – Paramedics*. London: HCPC.

Health and Care Professions Council (HCPC) (2016) *Standards of Conduct, Performance and Ethics*. London: HCPC.

Health and Social Care Information Centre (2014) *Code of practice on confidential information*. Available at: https://digital.nhs.uk/data-and-information/looking-after-information/data-security-and-information-governance/codes-of-practice-for-handling-information-in-health-and-care/code-of-practice-on-confidential-information.

Information Governance Review (2013) *Information: To Share or Not to Share*. Available at: https://assets.publishing.service.gov.uk/government/uploads/system/uploads/attachment_data/file/192572/2900774_InfoGovernance_accv2.pdf.

Parsa-Parsi, RW (2017) The Revised Declaration of Geneva: a modern-day physician's pledge. *JAMA*, 318(20): 1971–72.

United Nations General Assembly (1948) *Universal Declaration of Human Rights* (217 [III] A). Available at: www.un.org/en/universal-declaration-human-rights.

Warren, DN and Brandeis, L (1890) The right to privacy. *Harvard Law Review*, 4(5): 193-220.

UK Cases

Campbell v Mirror Group Newspapers [2002] EWCA Civ 1373

Furniss v Fitchett [1958] NZLR 356

Gillick v West Norfolk & Wisbech Area Health Authority [1986] AC 112

Hunter v Mann [1974] 1 QB 767

Hutchinson (Formerly KGM) v News Group Newspapers Ltd. [2011] EWCA Civ 808

Lady Archer v Williams [2003] EWHC 1670

Lewis v Secretary of State for Health [2008] EWHC 2196

R (on the Application of S) v Plymouth City Council [2002] EWCA Civ 388

R (Axon) v Secretary of State for Health [2006] EWHC 37

R v Mid-Glamorgan Family Health Services ex parte Martin [1995] 1 All ER 357

Viddal-Hall v Google Inc. [2015] EWCA Civ 311

W v Edgell [1989] EWCA Civ 13

X v Y [1998] 2 All ER 648

EU Cases

MS v Sweden [1997] ECHR 49

Z v Finland [1997] 25 EHRR 371

UK Legislation

Access to Health Records Act 1990

AIDS (Control) Act 1987

Care Act 2012

Children Act 1989

Criminal Law Act 1967

Data Protection Act 1984

Data Protection Act 1998

Data Protection Act 2018

Family Law Reform Act 1969

Health and Social Care Act 2001

Health and Social Care Act 2012

Human Rights Act 1998

Mental Capacity Act 2005

National Health Service Act 2006

Police and Criminal Evidence Act 1984

Prevention of Terrorism Act 2005

Public Health (Control of Disease) Act 1984

Road Traffic Act 1972

Road Traffic Act 1991

Terrorism Act 2000

Terrorism Act 2006

EU Legislation

Directive 95/46/EC

Directive 2002/58/EC

Directive 2006/24/EC

Regulation 2013/611

Regulation 2016/679

Legal and Ethical Considerations in the Use of Social Media

Aidan Baron

Introduction

Social media is a series of platforms that have significantly changed the way in which our society interacts. It has become a part of our daily lives and has created a more aware and conscious global community through the sharing of vast amounts of information. Whilst this globalisation can be an inherent source for 'good' in many cases, tensions also exist between social media and the professional responsibilities of registered professionals such as paramedics.

A benefit of social media is that it can promote the sharing of knowledge and experiences, often in real time. This feature can be particularly useful in major disasters, where social media has proven to be a vital tool for public health information dissemination (Simon et al. 2014). Social media has also contributed to an educational revolution in that it has allowed the sharing of knowledge amongst health practitioners from multiple disciplines around the world, where the Free Open Access Medical Education (FOAMed) concept has created a unique online community of practice (Roland et al. 2017). However, social media use can also pose risks both to paramedic users posting about incidents and those patients to whom the content of social media posts might refer.

This chapter will explore the unquestionable tension that rightfully exists between healthcare, where confidentiality and privacy are core tenets of practice, and social media, whose underpinning principle is to share. Drawing on ethical and legal arguments, consideration will be given to how social media can be used as a positive tool for good without compromising patients' privacy and trust in the paramedic service or the health service.

The Legal Obligations for Paramedics using Social Media

The use of social media by paramedics is governed by complementary layers of legislation, professional codes, policies and organisational guidelines. Personal information is protected under the General Data Protection Regulation (GDPR) of 2016 (Directive 95/46/EC), which explicitly specifies the rights of individual people and the responsibilities of organisations to protect these data. This superseded the Data Protection Act 1998, partly due to the complexity of the internet era. A chief focus of the GDPR is the role of technology and how data (which includes patient information in this context) is processed. Additionally, the UK is a human rights jurisdiction which recognises privacy as a human right (the Human Rights Act 1998) and a basic need 'essential to the development and maintenance both of a free society and of a mature and stable individual personality'.

These legal frameworks act in concert with professional codes and standards such as the Health and Care Professions Council's (HCPC) *Standards of Conduct, Performance and Ethics* (HCPC 2016), *Guidance on Social Media 2017* (HCPC 2017) and the *Standards of Proficiency – Paramedics* (HCPC 2014). Paramedic practice with regard to the use of social media should be informed not only by these laws, codes and guidelines, but also by professional body and employer policies, provided these are consistent with the law and regulatory body requirements (Baron and Townsend 2017).

Confidentiality and Social Media

Before the ancient Greek physician and philosopher Hippocrates, disease was believed by most people to be a form of punishment from divine beings. Hippocrates was one of the first recorded individuals to dispel this theory and suggest that it was a result of natural causes. Still, there remained an element of shame and social stigma surrounding most forms of disease which persists to this day. In his now-famous oath of the physician/healer, Hippocrates pledges: 'And whatsoever I shall see or hear in the course of my profession, as well as outside my profession in my [interactions with others], if it be what should not be published abroad, I will never divulge, holding such things to be holy secrets' (Conrad 1995).

Although many facets of the original Hippocratic Oath may now be outdated, the responsibility of the healthcare professional to preserve the confidentiality (privacy and secrecy) of this information remains a universal duty. As was outlined in Chapter 5, as a result of the development of society and its needs, there are now multiple mechanisms which govern what healthcare professionals, including paramedics, must and must not do, especially when it to comes to the sharing of information and the privacy of patients. The invention of the internet and its rapid growth has meant that at times these principles may appear not to apply. However, they continue to exist, and the onus is on the healthcare professional to ensure that they are aware of the way in which these principles can be applied and upheld when new technologies emerge.

Preserving a patient's confidentiality is important for several reasons. The most obvious reason confidentiality is so important is that patients can suffer significant psychosocial, financial and sometimes even physical harm when their private information is made public or falls into the wrong hands. This is recognised in many pieces of privacy law both in the UK and elsewhere that place a special privilege on personal health information. This is because health information is usually the most intimate type of information that an individual holds and may not even be shared with those closest to the individual. Paramedics are one of the few who are likely to be privy to the most intimate secrets of an individual and, as such, must take that privilege and the responsibility that accompanies it extremely seriously. As paramedics, we are given a great deal of trust by the patients whose crises we enter into, often in their homes or private places, and of whom we ask invasive questions about their lives, medical history, social histories and personal relationships. It is a legitimate fear for an individual that their privacy could be breached and that information they do not wish to share with others could be made public. Therefore, it is vital to preserve the public's trust in the ability of the entire profession to maintain confidentiality. If the public begins to distrust the ability of paramedics, both individually and as a whole profession, to preserve the privacy of their information, then it is very possible that members of the public will be less likely to call paramedics for help in a medical emergency. For this reason, behaviours which violate or breach the confidential nature of the relationship between the patient and a paramedic can not only harm that patient, but can also harm the professional reputation of all paramedics and the patients whom they might care for (see Chapter 2 for more details). Even a social media post which is actually lawful, but appears or can be perceived to be a breach of privacy can still cause real harm in this way.

Therefore, guidelines about the use of social media do not simply refer to the paramedic's duty to act lawfully; there is also a duty to act ethically to preserve not only the confidentiality of the patient, but also the patient's confidence in the profession and indeed all health professionals. This principle underpins the foundation of the healthcare practitioner regulatory scheme set out in the Health and Social Work Professions Order 2001, which recognises that trust and confidence by a patient in a professional is essential to the effective and efficient functioning of the healthcare system.

Ethical Considerations When Paramedics Use Social Media in a Professional Capacity

The paramedic profession is generally altruistic, with a professional duty to advocate for their patient and place their patient's interests above all else as part of their therapeutic relationship. It is unsurprising that ethical considerations merge with regulatory guidance when considering how social media can be used as a platform for 'good' by paramedics.

The HCPC expanded on its 2017 *Guidance on Social Media* (HCPC 2017) in October 2018, issuing a letter commenting that 'HCPC registrants' primary consideration should be their service user; raising the profile of their profession should only ever be a secondary consideration, and should not impact the service user's privacy or dignity. When live tweeting in order to raise the profile of the profession, registrants should take care to only share information required to achieve that objective. They should post in a modest manner; only providing the information the public needs to understand the role, and they should ensure any additional information, in particular service user identifiable information, isn't included' (HCPC 2018). This is an important explanation of the guidelines that have always existed but that, at times, have appeared to be unclear to some paramedics and ambulance services.

Good for the Public?

Individuals and organisations that appear to have abused their privileged position and to have breached their duty of confidentiality towards patients by posting on social media are often challenged by other professionals on social media from around the globe.

Pause for Thought

Chapter 3 discusses this ethical principle in more detail, and the reader may reflect on their perception of 'good' use of social media.

The reply to this challenge that is often cited is that publication of patient information is in the 'public interest' because it is posted by publicly funded organisations for the benefit of 'public education' in an effort to 'improve understanding of the role of paramedics' and 'decrease inappropriate use of ambulances' through 'service and profession promotion'. The paramedic and ambulance service tweeters approach this from a purely consequentialist approach, where an action is considered 'good' if, all things considered, the outcome or result is good. The promotion of an emergency service is a positive aspiration; however, the means by which this is accomplished should be healthily scrutinised and it often seems that the bad consequences are not accurately weighed up. One must remember that the entire purpose of the ambulance services is to care for those in crisis or in vulnerable situations and not to (ab)use the tragedy of others for the promotion of an organisation, whether that be a public institution or a charitable service.

There is a common misconception amongst paramedics that information and advice can be shared to improve public education as this is in 'the public interest'. However, as was outlined in Chapter 5, the use of any confidential information for the 'public interest' actually refers to a very specific legislative exemption from confidentiality provisions where the risk of breach of privacy of an individual is deemed to be less than the risk posed by not disclosing particular public health information to the wider community.

Public campaigns which cite the principles of narratives found within hermeneutics to discourage the use of pressured healthcare services have not yet been demonstrated to be effective. However, the tone of many of these posts often has the unintended consequence of maligning patients, commonly referred to as 'patient blaming'. This can be exceptionally damaging to the public perception of the profession and, indeed, the operating service, and also collides with the principles set out in Chapter 2 considering the professionalism offered by the registry body.

Tips for Practice

1. If a person can recognise themselves from something you post on social media, then it is unethical to post it without their permission.

2. Make it generalisable. When posting about an interesting case or learning point, wait at least a month, and change ages and genders.

3. Even private social media (such as closed Facebook groups) are not secure – discussing specific cases on these is not OK.

4. You cannot ask someone for consent to use their story or case during an emergency. You must wait until after that episode of care.

5. Use social media to hear directly from patients and find like-minded colleagues. It's a tool that can be used to share knowledge and ideas.

Social Media versus Television Documentary

Often a false equivalence is made between social media activity by ambulance services and paramedics, and television shows which feature real footage of ambulance calls and care of patients by paramedics. There is a crucial distinction that must be made between these two formats and that is the distinction of voluntary informed consent. When major broadcasting agencies produce television programmes which feature real-life footage of emergencies, they go through a rigorous process of obtaining voluntary informed consent from the patients and or family members being filmed, as well as the paramedics. This process involves not only seeking permission to film while an incident is occurring, but also going back to the patient and/or family afterwards (often months later) to seek actual written consent when that person(s) is not under the duress of an emergency situation. They do this so that there is no conflict of interest between those providing care (paramedics, who have additional responsibilities when compared with members of the public) and those doing the filming (the camera crew). The removal of the conflict between a treating paramedic and a patient is critical to ensure that the patient does not feel coerced into consenting to filming in exchange for getting access to good-quality care. If a paramedic were to make this request of a patient during or immediately after care, patients may feel obliged or pressured into granting consent for images or information to be shared, and this might not only represent a conflict to the paramedic, but may also pose a legal and ethical dilemma. This is clearly problematic on two fronts: first, from a utilitarian perspective, it can place the patient in an uncomfortable position (resulting in unhappiness); and, second, it calls into question whether the consent given is truly voluntary and informed (as discussed in Chapter 7).

Summary

In this modern era of the internet and globalisation, social media can be an inherent cause for 'good', but misuse can cause far-reaching mal-effects – for the patient, the paramedic and the profession. Ethical, lawful and beneficent use of social media by paramedics can be summarised as online behaviour which avoids referring to patients in any way, but instead focuses on education and public health promotion regarding diseases, advice, warning or communication relating to generic public circumstances. Using social media in this way avoids conflict of confidentiality, prevents misuse and continues to promote public trust in the profession and the services paramedics work within.

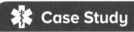 **Case Study**

At 21:30 on 6 April 2016, a 19-year-old female driver and her 16-year-old sister are involved in a major road traffic collision when their car hits black ice on the road and crashes into a tree beside the motorway. Local emergency services crews respond to the incident. An investigative journalist wants to find out what happened and so pieces together the following publicly available information using social media posts:

(continued)

06/04/2016 21:50 The local news broadcast posts on Twitter and Facebook

Two female passengers are being treated by Fakeshire ambulance and rescue crews after a major crash on the M75 motorway, closing down traffic in both lanes. Please drive safely.

06/04/2016 22:00 Fakeshire Ambulance Trust tweets:

Multiple crews have been dispatched to treat two young females involved in a major collision on the M75 motorway. Both have been transported to Fakeshire hospital in a critical condition. Remember to call 999 in an emergency.

06/04/2016 08:30 Sam Sun, official Fakeshire ambulance trust tweeter, tweets:

On the truck today with Stephanie Sticks, ready for a great week ahead.

06/04/2016 22:25 Fakeshire Air Ambulance Charity tweets:

Our advanced medical team attended a major RTC tonight. Two patients, one with major head and chest injuries. Thanks to our sponsors, we are able to deliver pre-hospital anaesthesia and blood products to those who need it most, saving lives in critical moments.

The accompanying Instagram post shows a picture of an incident, involving a car barely recognisable against a tree, multiple emergency service vehicles and blue lights. At the centre of the picture, the words 'Critical Care Doctor' and 'Critical Care Paramedic' are visible on the back of uniforms bending over what appears to be a patient, who is supine on the roadside.

06/04/2016 22:30 Melanie Smith, an official tweeter for Fakeshire Ambulance Trust, tweets:

Tough job tonight. First time doing a needle chest decompression this year. Big hugs to my emergency services family.

06/04/2016 22:40 Stephanie Sticks, not an official Fakeshire Ambulance Trust tweeter:

Thanks Fakeshire Air Ambulance and Fakeshire Fire and Rescue for all your help. Great teamwork as always tonight.

06/04/2016 23:30 Tim Chu, not an official tweeter for Fakeshire Ambulance Trust, but is tagged in a photo from the previous day with Melanie Smith where they are clearly seen as crewmates:

#MyEMSday

78yo asthma salbutamol neb-> A&E

65yo fall at home, referred to GP and falls team

16yo Head injury, RSI and thoracostomies -> MTC

21yo male, intoxicated and badly sprained ankle -> local MIU

07/04/2016 09:00 Sam Sun, official Fakeshire Ambulance Trust tweeter:

Remember that sometimes emotional shock can present in unusual ways. Catatonia, incontinence and paralysis can be psychologically induced from seeing a loved one being injured. Be alert.

What We Can Learn from This Case Study

The investigative journalist is able to piece together that the younger sister who is 16 years old has suffered a head injury and chest injuries, causing a tension pneumothorax requiring needle decompression, rapid sequence induction and blood product transfusion, and was then transported to Fakeshire major trauma centre. The second patient, the older sister who is 19 years old, likely also suffered an acute stress reaction which resulted in catatonia and urinary incontinence. This information, when pieced together, contains the age, injury pattern, treatments and clinical decisions made by paramedics for the patients whilst under their care. Such a level of detail should never be publicly available and is the private information belonging to the patient. Unfortunately, in this case, this highly sensitive and private information has now been made public. This is an example of how seemingly non-identifying or compromising pieces of information can, in combination, reveal a large amount about a person and incident.

Recommended Reading

Health and Care Professions Council (HCPC) (2017) *Guidance on Social Media*. London: HCPC.

Health and Care Professions Council (HCPC) (2018) *Social media in professional practice*. Available at: http://hcpc-uk.blogspot.com/2018/10/social-media-in-professional-practice.html.

References

Baron, A and Townsend, R (2017) Live tweeting by ambulance services: a growing concern. *Journal of Paramedic Practice*, 9(7). doi: 10.12968/jpar.2017.9.7.282.

Conrad, LI (1995) *The Western Medical Tradition: 800 BC to AD 1800*. Cambridge: Cambridge University Press.

Health and Care Professions Council (HCPC) (2014) *Standards of Proficiency – Paramedics*. London: HCPC.

Health and Care Professions Council (HCPC) (2016) *Standards of Conduct, Performance and Ethics*. London: HCPC.

Health and Care Professions Council (HCPC) (2017) *Guidance on Social Media*. London: HCPC.

Health and Care Professions Council (HCPC) (2018) *Social media in professional practice*. Available at: http://hcpc-uk.blogspot.com/2018/10/social-media-in-professional-practice.html.

Roland, D, Spurr, J and Cabrera, D (2017) Preliminary evidence for the emergence of a health care online community of practice: using a netnographic framework for Twitter hashtag analytics. *Journal of Medical Internet Research*, 19(7): p.e252.

Simon, T et al. (2014) Twitter in the cross fire? The use of social media in the Westgate Mall terror attack in Kenya. *PLoS ONE*, 9(8): p.e104136.

UK Legislation

Data Protection Act 1998

Data Protection Act 2018

Health and Social Work Professions Order 2001

Human Rights Act 1998

EU Legislation

Directive 95/46/EC

Chapter 7

Consent
Vince Clarke

Introduction

Paramedics, along with other healthcare professionals, usually need to make physical contact with their patients in order to assess, examine and treat them. The right to undertake such physical contact is limited in law and should only be done with the permission of the patient concerned. Such permission is termed 'consent'.

In some cases, the ability of the paramedic to obtain consent from a patient is interfered with, perhaps due to the clinical presentation of the patient (for example, if they are unconscious) or due to the circumstances in which the patient is presented, such as if they are in situations where family or friends may influence their decision making.

This chapter will set out what is meant by consent in relation to adult patients aged 18 and above, and will seek to clarify both the importance of gaining consent and the possible ramifications when appropriate consent is not gained. Consent in those under the age of 18 is discussed separately in Chapter 11.

What is Consent?

Consent can be considered simply as the giving of permission by a patient for a clinician to act. When considering medical ethics, Gillon (1994) defined consent as a voluntary, uncoerced decision, made by a sufficiently competent or autonomous person on the basis of adequate information and deliberation, to accept rather than reject some proposed course of action.

This is a seminal definition, and whilst the debates around the definition have progressed considerably since this was written, this definition offers the important underpinning features of consent.

Obtaining consent from patients is a central tenet of the special relationship between healthcare professionals and service users, and has legal, moral and clinical functions. Legally, the gaining of consent can protect the clinician from what might otherwise be considered to be unlawful touching. Morally, it is essential in order to fulfil the ethical duty of respect for autonomy. Clinically, the gaining of consent engenders co-operation and trust between the clinician and the service user, enabling an easier treatment experience for all parties.

Without gaining consent, any invasive medical treatment could amount to assault and/or battery. Patients who have capacity have the right to refuse to give consent to any assessment or treatment, even if their reasons may appear to the healthcare professional to be bizarre, irrational or non-existent. This right to refuse applies even if such a refusal might result in the death of the patient.

A Brief History of Consent

In the past, when the paternalistic approach of 'doctor knows best' was the mainstay of the medical profession, consent was something that was, on the whole, presumed. Doctors were not questioned, nor did they explain their actions or intentions to their patients. This approach began to change in the mid-twentieth century, when patients started to become both better informed and more litigious. This evolution coincided with developments in the field of medical ethics, the principles of which require patients to be placed in a position of greater control of their medical treatment (see Chapter 3).

Emphasis on the importance of consent was provided early in English law in *Beatty v Cullingworth* (1896), where the patient underwent surgery to remove one diseased ovary, but whilst under the anaesthetic, the surgeon found both ovaries to be diseased and removed both, without the tacit, verbal or written consent of the patient. Following on from this, it was advised that consent should be either in writing or in the presence of witnesses. From this point, various cases were seen within Britain and the USA, with perhaps one of the best known being *Schloendorff v Society of New York Hospital* (1914) and *Hunter v Burroughs* (1918). In the latter, as well as gaining consent, it was found that 'it is the duty of a physician in the exercise of ordinary care to warn a patient of the danger of possible bad consequences of using a remedy'. From these cases, the foundation for the legal application of consent in the medical setting was quite clearly established.

The 1957 case of *Salgo v Leland Stanford Jr University* saw the term 'informed consent' used for the first time, beginning a debate regarding the distinction between cases which could be brought alleging battery and those alleging a breach of duty, a matter that is further discussed later on in this chapter. The main focus of any litigious claim around consent was based on the degree of information that was shared with a patient, the basic principle being that had the patient known of the (undisclosed) risk, they would not have consented to the procedure.

In the UK, the cases of *Bolam v Friern Hospital Management Committee* (1957) in England and *Hunter v Hanley* (1955) in Scotland set the standard for what was considered to be 'reasonable' in respect of the amount of information expected to be given to a patient prior to their consent. Using the Bolam test when considering breach of duty is discussed separately in Chapter 8.

The Bolam test also stood as the standard in respect of consent until it was overruled in 2015, when the case of *Montgomery v Lanarkshire Health Board* was heard. In *Montgomery*, the test of materiality (what is material, or relevant, to be disclosed) was amended and moved on from the standard set in the Bolam test. The test of materiality defined in the *Montgomery* ruling was whether 'a reasonable person in the patient's position would be likely to attach significance to the risk, or the doctor is or should reasonably be aware that the particular patient would be likely to attach significance to it'.

Up to this point, using the Bolam test, it may have been the opinion of a doctor, and their peers, that it was reasonable, or in the best interests of a patient, to not disclose details of certain risks associated with a procedure in gaining consent to undertake the procedure. However, this position cannot be held following the *Montgomery* ruling.

Montgomery v Lanarkshire Health Board (2015)

Nadine Montgomery was a diabetic woman of small stature. She delivered her son vaginally, but he unfortunately experienced complications owing to shoulder dystocia, resulting in hypoxic insult which resulted in cerebral palsy. Montgomery's obstetrician had not disclosed the increased risk of this complication in vaginal delivery, despite her specifically asking if the baby's size could present a potential problem. Montgomery sued for negligence, arguing that if she had known of the increased risk, she would have requested a caesarean section instead of opting for a vaginal delivery. The UK Supreme Court judged in her favour in March 2015. This ruling overturned the previous decision made by the House of Lords in the case of Bolam, which had been law since the mid-1950s (Heywood 2015). It established that, rather than being a matter for clinical judgement to be assessed by professional medical opinion, a patient should be told whatever they want to know, not what the doctor thinks they should be told (Chan et al. 2017).

The nature of obstetric cases is such that they can be very complex and situations can change in a matter of moments. The ruling in *Montgomery* is likely to have the greatest impact on such cases, where the 'what if' discussions between the patient and the obstetrician whilst gaining consent will need to be particularly thorough and based on an individual patient's needs, following the guidelines already in place by the General Medical Council (GMC) (2008).

A non-obstetric example of the application of the *Montgomery* ruling can be found in *Spencer v Hillingdon Hospital NHS Trust*. In this case, the patient had consented to a hernia operation. After the operation, he suffered from bilateral pulmonary emboli. Because he had not been advised of the risk of deep vein thrombosis or pulmonary embolism, or of symptoms that might indicate these, he did not seek immediate treatment. The judge considered the *Montgomery* ruling and found that failure to inform the patient of the risks as part of the consent-gaining process was a breach of duty of care (Chan et al. 2017).

The outcome of this case is unlikely to have any direct impact on the practice of paramedics within the ambulance service, whose assessments and treatments are most commonly undertaken in unplanned situations that are urgent or emergency presentations with limited alternatives available. As paramedics continue to move into other settings, it becomes more relevant to consider the ruling in *Montgomery*. However, professional guidance promoting best practice would always seek to involve the patient in their care decisions, so any overt changes to practice are not likely to be seen. Indeed, the ruling in *Montgomery* was seen by a number of commentators to simply recognise the professional guidance regarding consent which had already been in place for a number of years (Chan et al. 2017).

What Makes Valid Consent?

As alluded to by Gillon (1994) above, in order to be considered valid, consent relies on three factors:

- The patient must have capacity.

- Consent must be given voluntarily.

- The nature of the proposed treatment must be understood, in broad terms, by the patient.

Each of these areas will now be briefly explored.

Capacity

As discussed in Chapter 3, autonomy is a fundamental ethical right of patients. Treatment can only be undertaken with consent, otherwise a patient's autonomy will have been ignored. The result is that a patient with capacity can lawfully refuse to give their consent to a proposed treatment. If this is the case, then the clinician who goes against the wishes of the patient can find themselves liable for battery. In cases where the adult patient lacks capacity, there is a requirement to act in the best interests of the patient. The matter of capacity will be further explored in Chapter 10, but it is important to note that consent, or the refusal of consent, *cannot be valid without capacity.*

Voluntariness

Consent is only valid when it is given voluntarily. The nature of medical consent is such that the circumstances in which it is sometimes sought (such as in life-threatening situations) may result in the degree of voluntariness being adversely affected. There are three main elements to be considered when judging the voluntariness of a patient's decision: coercion, undue influence and mistake.

Coercion

Coercion occurs where one party successfully and intentionally influences another by presenting a credible threat of unwanted and avoidable harm so severe that the person is unable to resist acting in order to avoid it. Acts of coercion are often seen in abusive relationships where the abusive partner controls the actions of the abused by controlling their behaviour. This type of controlling or coercive behaviour in intimate or familial relationships was made a specific offence in England and Wales as part of section 76 of the Serious Crime Act 2015, later replicated in Northern Ireland and Scotland. If there is any suspicion that a patient is being coerced into a decision regarding their treatment, the patient may need to be considered a vulnerable adult and this would need to be reported through the appropriate local channels. Coercion is less likely to be encountered than undue influence.

Undue Influence

Undue influence is not the same as persuasion. In many clinical contexts, the clinician is undertaking to persuade a patient to agree to a particular course of treatment because it is considered by the clinician to be in the patient's best interests. The act of persuasion usually involves giving a greater amount of information, and supporting evidence, to enable the patient to make an informed decision. This makes it distinct from undue influence.

Undue influence can, in law, be presumed in situations where the relationship between the patient and the persuader is one where there is an actual or perceived imbalance of power. For example, a parent can be presumed to have undue influence over their child, or an employer over an employee. Persuasive arguments where an imbalanced power relationship exists may be found to constitute undue influence. This was found to be the case in *Re T (Adult: Refusal of Treatment)* (1993), where a mother was found to have unduly influenced her daughter's decision-making process (although this was not the only material factor in the decision).

Re T (Adult: Refusal of Treatment) (1993)

The patient, T, was an adult female who was pregnant and had been involved in a road traffic collision. T consented to an operation to manage her internal bleeding, but had refused a blood transfusion following discussions with her mother, a Jehovah's Witness. T was not herself a Jehovah's Witness. Following that refusal, T's condition deteriorated and her baby was stillborn. T's father, supported by her boyfriend, applied for a declaration that it would be lawful to give her a blood transfusion. It was found by the court that there was no binding refusal and that blood could be lawfully administered in the best interests of T. On appeal, the Court of Appeal held that T's refusals were invalid due to both her incapacity and because they did not cover the extreme situation that had arisen. The undue influence of the patient's mother was also cited as leading to the invalidation of the refusal to consent to treatment.

As with most cases involving consent, T's was a matter of *refusal* to consent to treatment. Had the persuasive influence of her mother resulted in an agreement to the life-saving treatment recommended by the medical team, it is unlikely that a claim of undue influence would have been made by the doctors or other family members. This case demonstrates that the key consideration for paramedic practice is to consider the role of any third parties in the decision-making process of their patients.

Mistake

A mistake may occur where there is a material misunderstanding or a change of circumstances. In the case of *Re T*, discussed above, the initial refusal was informed in part by assurances that a blood transfusion might not be necessary and other alternative treatments could be used. As T's condition deteriorated, this was no longer the case, casting doubt on the validity of the initial refusal of consent. Mistake in this context is less likely to influence the validity of consent in cases involving paramedics.

Understanding the Proposed Treatment

Obtaining consent in paramedic practice presents a number of different challenges when compared to the medical profession. Medical doctors and surgeons often propose treatment that will be elective and undertaken at a point later in time relative to the gaining of consent. Therefore, there is sufficient time for a patient to gather the necessary information to become 'informed', either from the doctor or by their own means. The expectation of the patient to behave in a 'reasonable' manner in respect of their treatment is also a relatively recent development in the case law regarding consent.

> ### *Pause for Thought*
>
> *A (hypothetical) example might be a patient who is partially sighted and is undergoing a surgical procedure on their right shoulder. The 0.01% chance of sensory deficit in the fingertips associated with this procedure would not normally be considered by the profession to need to be shared with a patient undergoing this operation due to the extremely low incidence. For this patient, however, the loss of sensation in their fingertips would have a direct impact on their ability to read Braille. The relevance of this risk is therefore greater in the context of this patient.*

Previously, the degree of information that was expected to be shared by a clinician in order to represent the gaining of 'informed' consent was based on the opinion of the profession itself. The case of *Montgomery v Lanarkshire Health Board* (2015) moved this position by finding that there was a patient component within the informed aspect of consent, with individual patients requiring differing degrees of information based on their particular circumstances.

The 0.01% chance of sensory deficit in the fingertips associated with this procedure is information which the profession would not normally consider necessary to share with the patient undergoing the operation due to the extremely low incidence.

The test of informed consent is not necessarily that the patient would have refused to have the treatment if they had been informed of the associated risks, but rather that such information might be used by them to better prepare for such an outcome and be better informed prior to the procedure.

The risks associated with completing clinical observations, such as a pulse check, respiratory assessment or blood pressure reading, are so minimal as to require the lowest threshold of informed consent. Of these examples, only blood pressure assessment may cause some direct discomfort to the patient. The 'harm' brought about must be balanced against the 'benefit' of gaining a blood pressure reading, following the principles of ethical clinical practice (see Chapter 3). By explaining to the patient that they may feel some discomfort during the procedure, but that it is necessary in order for an appropriate clinical decision to be made about their care, the requirements of 'informed consent' have been met. The patient may then present their arm or pull up their sleeve in order for the blood pressure measurement to be undertaken. This action is sometimes considered as being 'implied consent', but, as has been demonstrated above, it is also appropriately informed.

Where the assessments become more invasive, such as a blood sugar reading or taking of blood samples, the potential risks should be shared with the patient. Again, the risks associated with these procedures are extremely minimal and would not require an in-depth, prolonged discussion.

Information regarding treatment and interventions should be more obviously considered and shared with the patient. The risks associated with the majority of paramedic interventions are set out by way of contraindications or cautions with procedures or medications. Ensuring that all information is shared with the patient prior to administering any medication or undertaking a procedure should appropriately cover all aspects of 'informing' in respect of consent to specific, potentially life-saving treatments. Challenges tend to arise in the lower acuity situations, where there are several possible treatment pathways available to a patient. Information is key to supporting a patient in making the decision that is right for them and therefore meets the expectations of informed consent.

Clearly, when a patient is unresponsive, consent cannot be gained in the same way as described above. This should not be seen as negating the need to consider how the patient should be informed – they may be unable to respond, but they may be able to hear what is being said and such a dialogue may reassure them. Additionally, discussing proposed assessments and treatments aloud informs any relatives or bystanders of what is being done and why, reducing any chance of misunderstandings which may lead to complaints of impropriety.

Tips for Practice

Patients must be given sufficient information to be able to decide what treatment they want to agree to and what treatment they want to refuse. The information should always be given in a way that the patient is able to comprehend, using appropriate language which the person understands.

Any information provided should address:

- the nature of the injury or illness, including its severity
- the nature of the proposed treatment and its purpose

(continued)

- any risks or side-effects associated with the proposed treatment which the person would find materially relevant

- any alternative approaches, including doing nothing

- the principle risks and benefits of the treatment, and any anticipated consequences.

The following potential challenges should also be considered:

- Information framing can be confusing, e.g. when explaining the odds of an adverse impact of treatment as being '1 case in 1,000' or as the same risk being '0.1%'. Be honest about clinical uncertainty.

- Medical complexity: as much information as the patient needs should be provided, with procedures explained to the level of detail they require, avoiding jargon and acronyms.

- A patient's illness may impact on their decision-making ability. Clinicians should show patience and give as much support as practicable.

- Being a patient can be disempowering. Patients should be supported to make their own decisions by the sharing of information.

Consent in the Emergency Setting

Valid consent must be sought and gained in all circumstances. However, gaining consent is not always possible in an emergency. Having established the core principles of consent, these now need to be applied with the consideration that the majority of paramedics work within an emergency and unscheduled care environment.

There are some exceptions when it may be permissible to provide care or treatment without explicit consent:

- When a person is not able to provide consent in an emergency and treatment is needed to save their life.

- Where a person has been assessed under the Mental Health Act 1983 as unable to consent to medical treatment due to a significant mental health disorder that affects their decision-making capability.

- Where a person is a risk to public health from a serious communicable disease.

Pause for Thought

Unrelated physical disorders still require the person to consent to treatment where they have capacity.

Patients who lack capacity, either through pre-existing conditions or through their being unconscious as a result of an acute illness or accident, should be treated in their best interests by adopting the *doctrine of necessity*. In an emergency, a patient may be treated without consent under the doctrine of necessity as long as there is a necessity to act when it is not practicable to communicate with the patient and that the action taken is no more than is immediately necessary in the best interests of the patient. This common law approach has been enshrined within the Mental Capacity Act 2005, and Chapter 10 focuses on patients whose capacity is diminished. In such cases, consent can be considered to be 'implied'.

The notion of 'immediately necessary' is not often a challenge for paramedics, where the extent and scope of their treatment will be limited to such interventions. Challenges in respect of consent and, more often, the refusal of consent tend to arise later in the hospital setting, where additional information and options become available. An example of such a situation is that of *Re AK (Medical Treatment: Consent)* (2001). In this case, AK was known to have motor neurone disease and that this degenerative disease would eventually result in his being unable to communicate or to move at all. An advance decision was put in place which specified that AK's life support ventilator be switched off two weeks after he lost the ability to communicate.

The challenges associated with advance decisions will be explored further in Chapter 10, with those related to end-of-life decisions considered in Chapter 12.

Consent and Mental Capacity

Mental capacity legislation across the UK is discussed in Chapter 10; however, it is important to briefly outline where consent and mental capacity legislation overlaps.

The Mental Capacity Act 2005 (for England and Wales) makes it clear that a person is presumed to be competent, with an ability to consent, until it is proven otherwise. If they cannot consent, a decision can be made in their best interests on their behalf. Section 27 of the Act lists some things that cannot be consented to on behalf of a person lacking capacity; however, it is unlikely that a paramedic in any role would be required to be involved with these.

Part 5 of the Adults with Incapacity (Scotland) Act 2000 allows treatment to be given to safeguard or promote the physical and mental health of an adult who is unable to consent. Special provisions apply where others (such as those with a power of attorney) have been appointed under the Act with powers relating to medical treatment. This Act also permits research involving an adult incapable of giving consent, but only under strict guidelines.

In Northern Ireland, the treatment of a patient lacking capacity is now governed by the Mental Capacity Act (Northern Ireland) 2016. Rather than providing legal powers to act, this Act is framed to protect the individual (such as a paramedic) from both civil and criminal liability when carrying out an act in the patient's best interests after determining that the patient lacks capacity to make a decision and so cannot consent. In general, this legislation outlines additional safeguards that need to be in place before a defined intervention is implemented.

What Can Happen if Appropriate Consent is Not Given?

There are some potentially misleading terms associated with consent – for example, when 'informed consent' is discussed as being different from 'implied consent'. In the context of inserting an intravenous cannula, for example, it is sometimes considered that the fact that a patient presented their arm when asked to do so represents 'implied consent' to the procedure.

Any form of consent must be valid, based on the three principles previously outlined. In cases where a patient has capacity, it could be argued that the paramedic saying 'I just need to pop a needle into your vein' and the patient presenting their arm does not constitute gaining appropriate consent. The consent 'implied' by the presentation of their arm does not represent an understanding of the potential risks associated with the procedure or the risks of not undergoing the procedure.

In the absence of a discussion regarding the clinical requirement to administer a drug by the intravenous route, the act of cannulation could be seen as an act of battery. Whether or not such an allegation arises depends to a large degree on the outcome of the procedure. If the patient were to develop an infection at the venepuncture site and suffer harm as a result, then there may be a case for a claim in negligence.

Consent must, by definition, be informed. Consent without information is not valid. However, the level of information that is required differs depending on both the intervention and the patient. In all cases of conscious adults with capacity, the aim should therefore be to gain appropriately informed consent for any assessment or intervention. Specific consent does not normally need to be sought in order to ask clinical questions and gain a history, with the responses of the patient effectively demonstrating consent to participate in the dialogue. In the case of patients who refuse to answer questions, the importance of their responding, from a clinical perspective, should be shared with the patient to ensure that they are fully aware of the consequences of not giving the information required to make a sound clinical decision in their treatment.

Consent and Criminal Law

Although it is suggested above that the gaining of consent can protect against prosecution for assault or battery, it does not offer a defence against the infliction of actual or grievous bodily harm. This is an area which will generally fall outside of the remit of the paramedic or ambulance clinician, whose invasive procedures are minimal, but is instead aimed at surgeons who undertake much more invasive procedures. For public interest reasons, such procedures are more often seen to sit outside of the criminal law and are accepted as being legally undertaken and termed 'reasonable surgical interference' (*Attorney General's Reference (No 6 of 1980) (1981)*). However, it is sometimes found that the 'surgical interference' undertaken is not considered 'reasonable' (*Devi v West Midlands RHS* (1980)). The limitations of the use of consent as a more general, non-medical defence are based on cases involving severe sadomasochistic practices where causing actual bodily harm is still considered an offence despite the 'victim's' apparent consent to such acts, such as in *R v Brown* (1993).

Devi v West Midlands RHS (1980)

Ms Devi was a 29-year-old female who consented to undergo an abdominal operation. This was to repair a perforated uterus which had been punctured following complications after the birth of her fourth child. During the operation, the surgeon carried out a hysterectomy, believing it was in Ms Devi's best interests to do so. The court found the surgeon liable for battery, as there was no consent given for the removal of the uterus.

Consent and Civil Law

Gaining consent broadly prevents a clinician from being liable in the civil courts for the tort of battery. This means that, provided the patient consented to treatment, there can be no possibility of an action to recover damages for 'unlawful touching'. However, this does not mean that there cannot be a claim in negligence if the consent given, or withheld, is found to have not been sufficiently informed, as was differentiated in *Chatterton v Gerson* (1981).

In cases concerning paramedics, it is commonly alleged that the attending clinician negligently failed to appropriately inform the patient of the possible adverse outcomes of refusing transport to hospital and subsequent assessment and treatment. The breach of this duty is more often found to lie in the clinical decision-making process of the paramedic, in that they did not recognise the potential adverse outcomes of a presenting complaint, rather than the position in the majority of claims made against surgeons, where they were aware of the risks but failed to disclose them (see *Chester v Afshar* (2004)). Chapter 8 will explore clinical negligence in much more depth.

Chatterton v Gerson (1981)

Mrs Chatterton underwent a hernia operation, a result of which was a trapped nerve that caused her severe pain. A pain specialist, Dr Gerson, performed an operation to relieve the pain, but this resulted in permanent immobility of her right leg. Mrs Chatterton said that she should have been informed of this risk and claimed battery. It was held that she had been informed in broad terms of the nature of the procedure, i.e. she had been informed and consented to an operation to her right leg. The fact that she may not have been informed of the specific risks of paralysis to her leg could not amount to battery; any claim would have to be made in negligence.

Chester v Afshar (2004)

The claimant, Ms Chester, was left partially paralysed following surgery for lumbar disc protrusion. Paralysis was a foreseeable but unavoidable risk of the surgery, with a risk of between 1% and 2%. Dr Afshar, the surgeon in the case, had failed to warn Ms Chester of this particular risk. The House of Lords concluded that whilst failure to warn of this risk was not a direct cause of the injury, it amounted to negligence. The comments made by Lord Bingham in the judgement appear to go beyond the Bolam test and lay the foundations for the later findings in *Montgomery*: 'A surgeon owes a general duty to a patient to warn him or her in general terms of possible serious risks involved in the procedure . . . In modern law medical paternalism no longer rules and a patient has a *prima facie* right to be informed by a surgeon of a small, but well-established, risk of serious injury as a result of surgery.'

What Form Should Consent Take?

Consent should be considered as a process rather than a one-off event: patients may change their minds or consent to one procedure, but not another. It is important to remember that consenting to, or requesting, a specific aspect of care or treatment does not imply consent to any other aspect of care.

The process of gaining consent is rarely recorded in writing, unless for specific surgical procedures; more often, it is a refusal of consent that is recorded on clinical documentation. There are very rarely any cases brought against ambulance clinicians or paramedics on the basis of consent where an assessment or treatment is actually carried out. The vast majority of litigation cases involve consent in the context of an absence of information being shared with the patient in order for them to make an informed decision regarding their consent to a particular treatment pathway.

Refusal of Consent to Treatment

Some cases are brought against paramedics where the nature of the information that they have given the patient leads that patient to 'refuse' consent (such as consent to transport to hospital) rather than a refusal of consent to assessment and treatment. Sometimes, the information that sways a patient's decision is related to perceptions of lengthy waiting times at hospital. While it may be appropriate to share such information, it is always the responsibility of the paramedic to appropriately inform their patient about the clinical ramifications of any decision to refuse treatment or further investigations.

It must be remembered that the patient is not a clinician and therefore is not in a position to make a clinical judgement. Cases where a paramedic starts a sentence with 'We could take you to hospital if you want, but. . .' are wholly inappropriate. If there is a clinical need for a patient to attend hospital or to be referred to an alternative care pathway, then this is the information that must be shared. It is rare for anyone to *want* to go to hospital when it is not necessary.

Refusal to consent to transport to hospital should be distinguished from refusal to receive treatment and also from refusal 'against advice'. Where the advice of the paramedic is that the patient should attend hospital, then that information and the rationale behind it must be clearly articulated to the patient and recorded within the documentation records.

Tips for Practice

- A signature is only evidence that the patient has signed the form; it is not proof of valid consent or informed refusal.
- If a patient is refusing treatment or transport, ensure that the information shared with them is accurately and fully recorded on any patient documentation.
- Where possible, ensure that your discussions with the patient are witnessed by a third party, whose details should be recorded on the appropriate documentation.

Summary

The gaining of consent from patients is a fundamental principle of healthcare. Although there may be challenges regarding the degree of information which should be shared to meet the expectations of the courts, the role of the paramedic is such that they are unlikely to fall foul of the law based solely on a matter of consent.

 Case Study 1: An Informed Refusal?

Michael is a 64-year-old man who lives alone. His past medical history includes a stroke two years ago and atrial fibrillation (AF), for which he takes rivaroxaban.

Michael was walking through his kitchen when he tripped and fell to the floor, hitting his head on the edge of the fireplace. He is a little shaken and has a 2.5 cm haematoma to his left temple. He did not lose consciousness and has no symptoms of a head injury. He attends the local minor injury unit and does not want to attend the emergency department.

The paramedic working within the unit informs Michael that whilst it is up to him, they would recommend that anyone who hits their head should go and get checked over in the emergency department to be on the 'safe side'. They do not doubt his capacity to make the decision for himself.

After returning home, Michael's friend visits later that day and finds Michael unconscious in a collapsed state on the floor. Michael is taken to hospital, where he later dies as a result of a brain haemorrhage.

(continued)

Question: Was Michael's refusal a valid refusal of consent?

Discussion: Considering the three requirements of valid consent, Michael had capacity to make the decision and the decision was made voluntarily. However, he was not sufficiently informed in order to make a decision.

Based on Michael's own particular circumstances, the general advice that minor head injuries do not require hospital assessment does not apply. Although the head injury is apparently minor, he is on an anticoagulant drug which increases his risk of intracranial haemorrhage, and this cannot be excluded outside of the hospital.

The matter of an invalid refusal of consent may apply if the paramedic was aware of this increased risk and failed to disclose it. It is more likely that the paramedic did not consider this risk and their clinical decision making fell below the reasonable standard expected of a paramedic, resulting in a breach of their duty of care.

Case Study 2: Another Refusal

Paramedics have been called to Paul, a 68-year-old male, who is experiencing chest pains. The 12-lead ECG clearly shows an ST elevation myocardial infarction. Paul has capacity and is refusing to travel to hospital.

Question: What information should be shared with Paul to ensure that the refusal is valid?

Discussion: It is most important that Paul knows that his presentation is potentially life-threatening. This should be set out in clear and simple terms which he can understand. The implications of not attending hospital, and the nature of any potential deterioration, should be explained. The method of treatment that the hospital may undertake should be discussed, along with the potential that this treatment would have to successfully treat Paul's condition. Clearly, only broad information can be given in this regard, as the paramedic cannot be expected to be fully conversant with all of the risks associated with a surgical intervention.

It should also be clear what Paul is refusing – either travel to hospital or treatment (or both). In the above scenario, Paul is refusing transport. This is different from refusing treatment. It may be the case that Paul wants to be treated for his presentation, but has his reservations about travelling to hospital. In some cases, this is due to something as simple as worrying about a pet that will be left alone if the patient is conveyed to hospital. Thoroughly exploring the patient's situation and gathering as much information as possible, both clinical and otherwise, will enable the paramedic to share sufficient, appropriate information to support the patient's decision making.

If, having shared all of this information, Paul still refuses to travel to hospital, then all of the information shared must be documented, and local procedures for non-conveyance adhered to.

Case Study 3: Refusal

Paramedics have been called to Julia, a 46-year-old female, who has fallen from her bed and spent the night on the floor. She is morbidly obese and has been lying on her left leg, which is now cold and blue. Julia has capacity and is refusing to travel to hospital against the clinical advice of the paramedic.

Question: What information should you record on your paperwork?

Discussion: All clinical findings and capacity test findings should be recorded as a matter of course. It is important to clearly document the information that has been given to Julia to assist in her decision-making process and, where possible, to record the reasoning expressed by the patient for refusing to give consent to treatment.

In such cases, arrangements should be made for a formal referral to the patient's own GP for follow-up assessment and treatment. Clinical documentation can inform both the patient and subsequent attending healthcare professionals, as well as protecting the attending paramedic.

 Case Study 4: Informed History-Taking

An ambulance has been called to Bob, a 56-year-old man, who has been experiencing sudden onset central chest pains. It is determined that Bob is suffering from acute coronary syndrome – treatment with aspirin and GTN is prepared. As per usual practice, the paramedic checks the contraindications to aspirin and GTN with Bob. Bob seems unsure when asked if he has taken sildenafil. The potentially life-threatening implications of administering GTN if Bob has taken sildenafil are explained. Bob acknowledges these risks and denies having taken sildenafil. GTN is administered and Bob promptly collapses due to a sudden reduction in blood pressure.

It transpires that Bob had taken sildenafil, but was too embarrassed to tell the paramedic.

Question: Does Bob have grounds for a claim in negligence?

It is unlikely that Bob could successfully sue for negligence. There is an expectation of the 'reasonable patient' as much as there is of the reasonable paramedic. It is likely that a judge would determine that the reasonable patient would, having been told of the risks associated with GTN administration, have refused consent based on their having taken sildenafil.

Recommended Reading

Lynch, J (2010) *Consent to Treatment*. London: CRC Press.

References

Chan, SW et al. (2017) *Montgomery* and informed consent: where are we now? *BMJ*, 357: j2224.

General Medical Council (GMC) (2008) *Consent: Patients and Doctors Making Decisions Together*. Manchester: GMC.

Gillon, R (1994) *Principles of Health Care Ethics*. Chichester: John Wiley & Sons.

Heywood, R (2015) RIP Sidaway: patient oriented disclosure – a standard worth waiting for. *Medical Law Review,* **23**(3): 455–66.

UK Cases

Attorney General's Reference (No 6 of 1980) [1981] QB 715

Beatty v Cullingworth (1896) QB Unreported 44 CENT LJ 153 (s896) 121

Bolam v Friern Hospital Management Committee [1957] 1 WLR 582

Chatterton v Gerson [1981] QB 432

Chester v Afshar [2004] UKHL 41 Pt 2

Devi v West Midlands RHS [1980] CLY 687

Hunter v Hanley [1955] SLT 213; [1955] ScotCS CSIH_2; 1955 SC 200; [1955–95] PNLR 1

Montgomery v Lanarkshire Health Board [2015] SC 11; [2015] 1 AC 1430

R v Brown (1993) 97 Cr App R 44; [1994] 1 AC 212

Re AK (Medical Treatment: Consent) [2001] 1 FLR 129

Re T (Adult: Refusal of Treatment) [1993] Fam 95

Spencer v Hillingdon Hospital NHS Trust [2015] EWHC 1058 (QB).

US Cases

Hunter v Burroughs, 13 June 1918 [96 SE 360]

Salgo v Leland Stanford Jr University Board of Trustees 154 Cal App.2d 560; 317 P.2d 170 (1957)

Schloendorff v Society of New York Hospital, 105 NE 92 (NY 1914)

Legislation: England and Wales

Mental Health Act 1983

Mental Capacity Act 2005

Serious Crime Act 2015

Legislation: Scotland

Adults with Incapacity (Scotland) Act 2000

Legislation: Northern Ireland

Mental Capacity Act (Northern Ireland) 2016

Chapter 8

Clinical Negligence

Edd Bartlett and Georgette Eaton

Introduction

In law, negligence is a tort, a 'civil wrong'. In order for a clinical negligence claim to be successful, the claimant needs to prove that three criteria have been met:

1. That the clinician owed the patient a duty of care.

2. That the clinician breached their duty of care.

3. That 'but for' that breach in duty, the patient would not have suffered harm.

These criteria apply to both adult and paediatric cases and across the whole of the UK. A claim in negligence is an understandable concern for all clinicians, with phrases such as 'if you didn't write it down, it never happened' often reinforcing litigious thoughts at the back of clinicians' minds when they are in training. Good quality documentation is, of course, essential to quality patient care, as well as important in the event of a claim in negligence. This chapter aims to ease some of the anxiety surrounding litigation by outlining the key concepts of a claim in negligence and highlighting the move towards a culture of learning from mistakes in the NHS.

Duty of Care

A duty of care is not a concept unique to medical negligence; it was established in the 1932 Scottish case *Donoghue v Stevenson*, known as the 'snail in the ale' case. A duty of care is established when it is reasonably foreseeable that a person's actions could cause either harm to another person or damage to their property.

Donoghue v Stevenson (1932)

The Facts of the Case

Mrs Donoghue drank a bottle of ginger beer which turned out to contain a dead snail. Following this, she became unwell and suffered 'severe gastroenteritis and shock'. She sued Mr Stevenson, who had manufactured the ginger beer.

The Judgement

The case went to the highest court at the time, the House of Lords, where it was ruled that Mr Stevenson had owed a duty of care to Mrs Donoghue and had not taken reasonable care to ensure that harm did not come to people who consumed his products.

In clinical negligence claims, the duty of care is normally easy to establish. In the hospital environment, it is established as soon as a person presents for treatment (*Barnett v Chelsea and Kensington Hospital Management Committee* (1969)). When a person calls 999 and asks for the ambulance service, this is when a duty of care is established (*Kent v Griffiths* (2000)). In the case of *Kent v Griffiths*, there was no reasonable excuse for the delay of the ambulance, which resulted in the patient, who was having an asthma attack, suffering a respiratory arrest followed by memory impairment and miscarriage. The judge ruled that the ambulance service had breached its duty of care and because of this breach had caused the patient harm.

Breach of Duty

In the law of tort, the test for breach of duty is: did the person act in a way that a reasonable person would have acted? The reasonable person is an average member of the public, often referred to as 'the man on the Clapham omnibus' (see Chapter 4).

In medical cases, a different test is used. A clinician must meet the standard of care that is expected from a skilled clinician. The standard of care that a health professional is expected to exercise is that of those in the speciality of the profession involved. A paramedic is to be assessed by the skills expected of a paramedic, not a GP (*Stockdale v Nicholls* (1993)). Therefore, a paramedic would not be negligent in failing to diagnose a condition that would only be apparent to a specialist in that field. However, a paramedic may be found negligent for not referring a patient with unusual symptoms for a follow-up appointment or secondary consultation (*Judge v Huntingdon Health Authority* (1995)).

Further, it would be negligent for a paramedic to attempt a medical procedure that should be attempted only by a specialist in that particular field (*De Freitas v O'Brien* (1993)). So, if a paramedic practises a skill that is not within their normal scope of practice (for example, suturing is a specialist and advanced skill), this will be judged against the standard of care expected of a reasonable clinician skilled in suturing. If they do not meet that standard, then they may be found to be negligent. This also means that if a person is acting in a particular capacity, then they must exercise the level of skill expected of such a person.

Inexperience (*Jones v Manchester Corporation* (1952)) is irrelevant as long as the person is deemed competent to perform a task expected of them within their specialism. However, an inexperienced member of staff may not be negligent in following the advice of a senior colleague. In *Wilsher v Essex Area Health Authority* (1986), a junior colleague was not found to be negligent for following the instructions of a senior colleague, who then subsequently checked the work. Despite this, a defence of 'only following orders' is not acceptable and first, the junior colleague must check their understanding of the instructions given by a senior colleague, and these instructions should not be blatantly wrong. A pharmacist who failed to confirm a prescription that was incorrect was found to be negligent (*Horton v Evans* (2006)). Interestingly, in *Antoniades v East Sussex Hospitals NHS Trust* (2007), the team leader was found to be negligent for having inadequately trained his team. This is an important consideration both for clinical team leaders as well as those working in education.

There are two main tests that are used to establish breach of duty: the Bolam test and the *Bolitho* test. In addition, clinical guidelines are increasingly being used to set the benchmark for a reasonable standard of care, although this does not mean they must always be adhered to (*C v North Cumbria University Hospitals NHS Trust* (2014)).

The Bolam Test

When care is delivered by any health professional, the standard of care expected is that of any reasonable health professional. The Bolam principle addresses the first element of breach of duty and summates that a health professional is not negligent if they act in accordance with a practice accepted at the time as proper by a responsible body of medical opinion.

Bolam v Friern Hospital Management Committee (1957)

Mr Bolam was a voluntary patient at Friern Hospital, a mental health hospital. He was prescribed electroconvulsive therapy (ECT) as a treatment for depression, but was not warned of any of the risks involved (such as convulsive shaking and risk of injury). He underwent the procedure without muscle relaxants or restraint. During treatment, he sustained a fractured hip and additional complications.

At the time, there was a division of medical opinion regarding the benefits of physical restraint and muscle relaxants during ECT, as well as the need to warn patients of the risk. Therefore, Mr Bolam failed to prove that the defendants had been negligent.

At the time of this case, medical negligence cases in England and Wales were decided by a jury. In his direction to the jury, McNair J (the judge) said that:

> A doctor is not guilty of negligence if he has acted in accordance with a practice accepted as proper by a responsible body of medical men skilled in that particular art.

Therefore, in situations which involve the use of some special skill or competence, the standard expected is not that of the ordinary reasonable man, but that expected by the ordinary skilled man who professes to have, and exercises, that special skill. Importantly, this test applies not only to doctors, but also any healthcare professional.

McNair J also added that a man 'is not negligent if he is acting in accordance with such a practice, merely because there is a body of opinion that takes the contrary view'. This has been taken to mean that even if a body of opinion does not agree with a professional's actions in given circumstances, if a body of opinion which did agree could be found, the professional would not be considered negligent.

However, in *Maynard v West Midlands Regional Health Authority* (1985), the House of Lords held that a judge is not in a position to choose between the views of competing medical experts. As long as there is a competent school of thought that supports the belief that the defendant's actions were reasonable, the judge will find the defendant not to have been negligent.

The effect of the Bolam decision is that it is difficult to show a doctor breached the duty of care: it is not about whether the defendant acted in the *ideal* way, but that their actions were above the minimal acceptable practice. Some of these criticisms of the Bolam test argue that doctors (or other health professionals) should not dictate whether conduct is negligent and that the court should more actively scrutinise the standard of care given.

Another issue is that the actual size of the body of medical opinion that Bolam requires is not explicit. In *De Freitas v O'Brien* (1995), expert evidence for the defendant showed that only a small number of peers would endorse the defendant's conduct, but Otton LJ states that the size of the medical body was less important than the fact that there was a *reasonable* body. This implies that the defendant's actions may be defensible even if there is only minority support.

Similarly, there can be a lack of objectivity. The Bolam test depends upon a body of medical opinion that endorses the defendant's practice. This could be based on a single expert, rather than evidence-based guidelines such as those from the National Institute for Health and Care Excellence (NICE). Objective evidence for clinical guidelines informed the outcome in *Richards v Swansea NHS Trust* (2007); however, this does not mean that a health professional who deviates from clinical guidelines will be negligent if something goes wrong. There is a danger in applying clinical guidelines rigidly in dynamic clinical situations, where they may not necessarily present 'best practice'. Nevertheless, the objectivity of the evidence-based guideline or the expert opinion used may in some situations impact on informing the standard of care expected. As was discussed in Chapter 7, the outcome of *Montgomery v Lanarkshire Health Board* (2015) means that the Bolam test cannot be held when gaining consent.

However, the law's approach is less clear-cut after the House of Lords' decision in *Bolitho v Hackney Health Authority* (1997).

Bolitho v Hackney Health Authority (1997)

Two-year-old Patrick Bolitho suffered brain damage during an attack of croup, leading to cardiac arrest. Evidence of the case accepted that the on-call paediatric registrar negligently failed to attend the patient and the question of causation concerned whether the attendance would have altered the outcome in any event. Expert witnesses were (unequally) divided and the decision was appealed to the House of Lords, which held that there needed to have been a logical basis for the decisions of the defendant and the expert witnesses.

The obiter comments of Lord Browne-Wilkinson provide an important understanding for how the court might adopt a more interventionalist approach when determining a standard of care. He referred to McNair J's comments in Bolam regarding the 'use of these adjectives – responsible, reasonable, and respectable – all show the court has to be satisfied that the exponents of the body of opinion relied upon can demonstrate that such an opinion has a logical basis'. In deciding whether the standard has been breached, the endorsement has to be from a source that can be relied upon and should have a logical basis that can withstand objective scrutiny. *Bolitho* indicates that it is not enough to have only opinion to support the practice in question and that the judge will need to scrutinise the evidence, especially in competing views.

Notably, many cases after *Bolitho* do not cite this 'second' measure and refer simply to the Bolam test. This in itself indicates that *Bolitho* and the comments of Lord Browne-Wilkinson may not have made as much of an impression as they probably should have. However, of the cases that have cited *Bolitho*, it does seem that this had a significant (if conflicting) impact on the scrutiny given to the expert opinion.

In *Marriott v West Midlands Health Authority* (1999), the trial judge (supported by the Court of Appeal) held that although a reasonable body of experts agreed with the actions of the defendant, such an approach was held to be irresponsible by the courts. This indicated that *Bolitho* authorises a judge to consider the views of medical experts, but also deems them irresponsible if appropriate.

In *Burne v A* (2006), the trial judge rejected the views of experts concerning what a reasonable course of conduct would be. However, at appeal, it was outlined that the judge should have done one or both of two things: to ask the claimant's counsel whether (should he or she find the expert evidence unacceptable) he or she should consider the credibility of the expert evidence in support of the doctor; and, if the claimant's counsel said yes, to ensure that the defendant's side had a proper opportunity to respond. Essentially, this case demonstrated that a judge could reject the views of experts on what is a reasonable course of conduct, but before doing so, the experts must be given the chance to justify practice.

Overlapping significantly with the law concerning mental health, in the case of *Border v Lewisham and Greenwich NHS Trust* (2015), a patient did not consent to the insertion of an intravenous line, but despite her mental capacity, this was undertaken. Whilst a body of experts believed the actions of the doctor had been appropriate, the Court of Appeal, citing *Bolitho,* found that treating a competent person against their wishes would be negligent.

Concerning *Bolitho,* if there is a conflict between experts, the judge must explain which expert is preferred and why (*Smith v Southampton University Hospital NHS Trust* (2007)) and it is not enough to only say that the expert is responsible alone (*Hanson v Airedale Hospital NHS Trust* (2003)). Ultimately, the judge should not simply accept expert opinion, and it should be tested for internal consistency and against the other evidence of the trial (*Mulholland v Medway NHS Foundation Trust* (2015)).

Mulheron (2010, pp. 637–38) outlines an excellent summary of the case law post-*Bolitho*, describing how to overrule medical practice under the Bolam test. If any of these points raise an answer in the negative, it constitutes a ground where English courts have previously rejected expert medical opinion as indefensible. The court should consider whether the expert evidence:

- took account of a clear and simple precaution which was not followed, but which, more probably than not, would have avoided the adverse outcome

- considered conflicts of duties among patients, and resource limitations governing the medical practice

- weighed the comparative risks/benefits of the medical practice, as opposed to other course(s) of conduct

- took account of public/community expectations of acceptable medical practice

- was correct in light of the factual context as a whole

- was internally consistent

- adhered to the correct legal test governing the requisite standard of care.

Whilst it is difficult to generalise from the small number of selected cases presented here, this discussion demonstrates that the courts are reluctant to abandon Bolam in respect of medical opinion, and that *Bolitho* is sometimes used as second 'back-up' position. Regardless of the criticism and the fact that these cases feature medical doctors, the point remains that these two main tests are used to establish breach of duty and determine negligence.

Causation

The final step to establishing a successful claim in negligence, and the stage at which many claims fail, is establishing causation. Causation requires that the breach of duty made a significant contribution to the harm caused to the patient. The test is commonly known as the 'but for' test: but for the breach in duty, no harm would have come to the patient. This is often complicated to prove as there can be multiple factors that affect a patient's outcome, the clinician's negligence being only one. In addition, the legal causation must be satisfied by the test for remoteness.

There are complex issues that can arise when the defendant is not shown definitely to have caused harm, but has been involved in the cause or exposed the claimant to risk. In *Barnett v Chelsea and Kensington Hospital Management Committee* (1969), a doctor refused to see a man who presented to the emergency department with abdominal pain and died shortly afterwards. Whilst it was clear that the doctor was negligent for refusing to see the patient, the evidence from the post mortem suggested that even if the doctor had seen the patient, the patient would have died from arsenic poisoning. This negligence did not cause the injury.

Causation may also be established from the 'loss of a chance', which is where but for the clinician's omission to offer treatment, the patient would on the balance of probabilities have made a recovery.

Hayes v South East Coast Ambulance Service (2015)

The Facts of the Case

Two ambulance technicians attended a 41-year-old brittle asthmatic (H), who presented as not being able to speak and having difficulty in breathing. They gave the patient one dose of salbutamol before walking him to the ambulance. They had only documented a blood sugar reading and Glasgow Coma Score. The crew did not give the patient ipratropium bromide or adrenaline; they also did not give any further doses of salbutamol. On the way to the ambulance, the patient suffered a respiratory and cardiac arrest, which resulted in his death.

The Judgement

The crew were found to be negligent:

- They had not identified that the patient's condition was life threatening.
- According to guidelines, he should have been given ipratropium bromide following the administration of salbutamol.
- Insufficient clinical observations were taken.
- They did not administer adrenaline.

It was found that, given the above: 'On the balance of probabilities, but for the negligent treatment, H would have survived . . . H's prospects of survival would have been 60 per cent' (paragraphs 137–141).

Hayes v South East Coast Ambulance Service demonstrates how the tests for negligence are applied:

1. There was a duty of care to the patient, which was established when H called 999, and the ambulance technicians had a duty of care when they were sent to the incident.

2. The breach of duty occurred when they failed to identify the severity of H's condition, did not take sufficient observations and failed to administer the drugs according to UK clinical practice guidelines (this would be measured against the guidelines that were being used at the time – JRCALC 2013 guidance). The Bolam test was applied and the opinion of an expert witness was sought. The expert witness, Dr Moore, confirmed that a reasonable technician would have recognised the severity of H's condition, taken suitable observations and administered the correct drugs.

3. Causation was established by the 60% chance that H would have survived but for the negligence of the attending crew.

After proving causation, the claimant must establish that the type of injury was not too *remote*: the type of harm must be a foreseeable consequence of the negligence. In clinical negligence situations, this can usually be shown.

Criminal Negligence

A criminal action can be brought in circumstances where the death of a patient is caused by the grossly negligent act or omission of a health professional. In *R v Adomako* (1995), the House of Lords held that criminal negligence can be found where the health professional – in this case, a doctor – is:

- indifferent about an obvious risk of injury to a patient

- aware of a risk, but decides to proceed in any event

- intending to avoid a known risk, but does so with a high degree of negligence

- inattentive or fails to be alert to a serious risk.

✳ Case Study

Maddy, a 29-year-old female, presents to a specialist paramedic in a busy urgent care centre. Maddy has lacerated her hand whilst washing up glasses in the sink. She is a jeweller, currently commissioned to design and make pieces for a well-known retail company. The laceration is across her right palm and she complains of slight numbness to the fingers as well as an inability to move her fingers well. She is worried this may impact on her job.

The specialist paramedic has recently joined the urgent care centre, having completed his portfolio of competencies. He looks at the wound, seeing that it is quite deep to the tendons, but notes that there is no neurovascular tenderness distal to the injury and there is active, passive and resisted range of movement in Maddy's fingers and wrist. He thinks the wound is suitable for suturing and proceeds to irrigate the wound, remove any remaining glass and meticulously suture the wound closed. He has never performed this procedure to the hand before, but has read about suturing palms in the past, and the unit team leader is already attending to a complex patient and so he goes ahead. He informs Maddy of worsening advice concerning infection or poor healing to the hand and discharges her home. He documents his care and later discusses the case with the unit team leader, who felt that his actions were appropriate.

Three weeks later, Maddy is concerned that the movement of her fingers is not back to normal and there is still some numbness present. She has been finding it difficult to perform the fine motor skills her work requires. She seeks an emergency appointment with a GP, who notes that she cannot bend three of her fingers partially or fully and that there is altered sensation present in two of these fingers. He sees the wound on her hand and she explains that this was caused by glass. The GP refers her to the hand clinic, where she was seen the following day.

At the clinic, a flexor tendon injury is determined, with some glass embedded in the wound, and the tendon is repaired under general anaesthetic. Maddy is put in a splint for six weeks and is unable to finalise the design for the commission she was working on. Despite hand therapy, three months later she still has not regained full motor movement in her hand and she subsequently loses her employment.

Evidence suggests that if Maddy had had an X-ray to determine the presence of glass in the wound and an immediate referral to the hand surgeon for assessment, her flexor tendon injury would have been spotted and repaired more quickly and she would have had a 40% chance of full recovery. The delay meant that the chances of having full movement of her fingers to undertake her employment were reduced to 5%.

As an 'expert witness', what advice would you give Maddy?

Problems with the Current System

While clinical negligence claims against the NHS have fallen by over 10% in the past three years, the cost of these claims are increasing, with the legal costs for lower-value claims sometimes exceeding the damages by three times (NHS Resolution 2017a, p. 8; 2017b, p. 12). NHS Resolution is working to reduce litigation and utilise more alternative dispute resolution solutions, such as mediation (NHS Resolution 2017b, p. 12).

The cost of clinical negligence claims is a substantial burden to the NHS and is one of the main focuses of criticism towards the current system. In 2015/16, 36% of £1.5 billion legal costs to the NHS were directly related to the cost of litigation (Department of Health 2017, p. 5). Clinical negligence claims against the ambulance service accounted for 2% of the total value of clinical negligence claims in 2016/17 (NHS Resolution 2017a, p. 23).

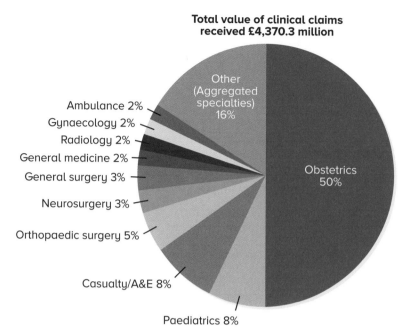

Total value of clinical claims received £4,370.3 million

Other (Aggregated specialties) 16%

Ambulance 2%
Gynaecology 2%
Radiology 2%
General medicine 2%
General surgery 3%
Neurosurgery 3%
Orthopaedic surgery 5%
Casualty/A&E 8%
Paediatrics 8%

Obstetrics 50%

Figure 8.1 Value of clinical negligence claims received in 2016/17 (NHS Resolution 2017a, p. 23)

Another criticism is that only compensating patients for injury caused by a medical error (a fault-based system) means that patients who suffer injury where no one is at fault receive no compensation (Douglas 2009). Douglas (2009, pp. 30, 36) gives three examples:

✴ Case Study

Case 1. Mr Smith suffers a brain haemorrhage as a result of a genetic defect in the arteries supplying his brain. He is taken immediately to hospital, where he is rushed to the operating theatre, unconscious, to have the blood drained from his skull. During the course of the operation, the surgeon negligently damages the part of his brain that controls his right leg. Though Mr Smith subsequently recovers from his haemorrhage, the damage inflicted by the surgeon leaves him with a permanently paralysed leg.

Case 2. Mrs Jones, like Mr Smith, suffers a brain haemorrhage as a result of a genetic defect. She too is rushed to the operating theatre and, as with Mr Smith, the surgeon damages the part of her brain that controls her right leg. In her case, however, the damage is not due to negligence on the surgeon's part. It is instead an unusual side-effect of good surgical practice: the surgeon (correctly) believes that it is necessary to damage this part of the brain in order to stop the haemorrhage and thus save Mrs Jones' life. However, the result is the same. Mrs Jones recovers from the haemorrhage, but is left with a permanently paralysed leg.

> *Case 3.* Mr Williams, like Mr Smith and Mrs Jones, suffers a brain haemorrhage as a result of a genetic defect. He too is rushed to hospital. However, his haemorrhage is particularly severe and before he can be taken to the operating theatre, the part of his brain which controls his right leg is irreversibly damaged. Thus, like Mr Smith and Mrs Jones, he is left with a paralysed leg, though in his case, the paralysis is a result of the genetic condition (and subsequent haemorrhage), not of its treatment.

Douglas (2009) points out that Mr Smith would have a successful claim in negligence, whereas Mrs Jones would not. In a fault-based compensation system, only Mr Smith would be compensated, which Mrs Jones may argue is unfair as she too suffered an injury from the surgery, albeit not as a result of negligence. However, in some jurisdictions, for example, New Zealand, she would receive compensation, as it operates a no-fault system.

A no-fault compensation system offers a person compensation regardless of whether their injury was caused by negligence. New Zealand's publicly funded compensation scheme, which was introduced in 1974 and reformed in 2005 to introduce a no-fault approach to medical error, provides patients with compensation for injury following medical treatment without the need to prove negligence (Wallis 2017).

Douglas points out that the no-fault system still does not provide compensation equality. What about Mr Williams from Case 3? He would not receive any compensation as his injury was caused by a natural occurrence. Douglas (2009) argues that a jurisdiction focusing on fair compensation for all who suffer illness or injury, from any cause other than self-infliction, should implement a system that compensates everyone equally. Douglas suggests that this could be achieved by moving away from a compensation system, be it fault or no-fault-based, and instead allow the broadening of social security and public healthcare systems to provide support to those who have suffered illness or injury, regardless of the cause (Douglas 2009, pp. 50–51).

In a fault-based system, in addition to worries about the cost of litigation against the NHS and compensation inequality, there are also concerns about the influence that the fear of litigation has on medical practice, meaning that clinicians may be afraid of owning up to errors.

> ### The Bristol Royal Infirmary Inquiry (2001, p. 366)
>
> *[T]he culture and the practice of clinical negligence litigation work against the interests of patients' safety. The system is positively counterproductive, in that it provides a clear incentive not to report, or to cover up, an error or incident. And, once covered up, no one can learn from it and the next patient is exposed to the same or a similar risk.*

In response to the Bristol Royal Infirmary Inquiry (2001) and Department of Health (2001) reports, a move towards open reporting was instigated. The National Patient Safety Agency (NPSA) was established and in 2003 the National Reporting and

Learning System was set up (NPSA 2018). This is a central database of over four million patient safety incident reports that is used by NHS Improvement to develop advice and guidance for the NHS, reducing risks to patients (NHS Improvement 2016).

NHS England (2015) has adopted a *Serious Incident Framework* that supports a no-blame approach to investigating incidents. Combined with the statutory duty of candour brought in by the Health and Social Care Act 2008 (Regulated Activities) Regulations 2014, this works towards the recommendations set out in the Francis Report of 'Openness, Transparency and Candour' (The Stationery Office 2013: 66).

Serious Incident Framework (NHS England 2015, p. 39)

Provider organisations should make it clear that the investigation itself is separate to any other legal and/or disciplinary process. Organisations must advocate justifiable accountability but there must be zero tolerance for inappropriate blame and those involved must not be unfairly exposed to punitive disciplinary action, increased medico-legal risk or any threat to their registration by virtue of involvement in the investigation process.

Despite the improvement in reporting and the move away from a blame culture since 2000, there remain concerns about the treatment of clinicians by the clinical negligence system. At the time of writing, this has been bought to the forefront of clinicians' minds by the case of Dr Bawa-Garba.

The details in *GMC v Bawa-Garba* (2018) demonstrate the complexity of decision making for seriously unwell children, as well as the consequences of medical error. In this case, a child was admitted to hospital with dehydration and subsequently died as a result of systemic sepsis. What is important to note from this case is that the clinician involved was experienced, knowledgeable and qualified for the role that was being undertaken. The child died, it is held, as a result of a delay in recognition and management of systemic sepsis by the admitting hospital.

In 2015, Dr Bawa-Garba, a specialist registrar in paediatrics, was found guilty of gross negligence manslaughter following the tragic death of Jack Adcock, a six-year-old with Down's syndrome, from septic shock (Dyer 2015). The treatment she provided was considered to be 'truly, exceptionally bad' as she failed to identify test results that indicated the patient's kidneys were failing and mistakenly stopped resuscitation efforts after mistaking him for another patient with a Do Not Resuscitate order. Although resuscitation was resumed after the error was identified, it was not successful and Jack was pronounced dead.

> **Pause for Thought**
>
> *In some cases, clinicians can be found to be so negligent that they are found to be criminally liable.*

In 2017, a Medical Practitioners' Tribunal decided it appropriate for Dr Bawa-Garba to be suspended from practice for 12 months and she was not removed from the medical register. This decision considered the 'multiple systemic failures' that contributed to the tragic events that day and Dr Bawa-Garba's 'unblemished record before and since along with evidence from colleagues and consultants who called her an excellent doctor' (Dyer 2017). The GMC did not agree with the decision of the Tribunal, believing that public trust could have been eroded by the decision, and in 2017, it appealed to the High Court to have Dr Bawa-Garba removed from the medical register, a move which was successful (*General Medical Council v Bawa-Garba* (2018)). Many doctors have raised concerns about the GMC's actions, believing that it endangers the national move towards an open and honest safety culture (Cohen 2017; Johannsson and Rook 2018).

Following a campaign that funded over £360,000 for her reinstatement, Dr Bawa-Garba appealed against the High Court ruling and the Court of Appeal rejected the High Court's decision. Dr Bawa-Garba was reinstated to the medical register in August 2018.

This incident happened in 2011 and a final ruling was issued in August 2018. Similar to the case of *Bolitho* (which occurred in 1984 and a final decision held in 1997), not only is paediatric clinical negligence complex, it can also take a significant amount of time to reach a final conclusion. In addition, the associated costs are high, as a child who suffers as a result of medical error in early life will need to be supported for as long as is necessary, which may be the rest of their life.

The double tragedy of Jack Adcock's death and Bawa-Garba's prolonged journey within the criminal justice system has shaken the medical and its associated professions. However, this has been a watershed moment in patient safety, which has highlighted critical issues within hospitals of understaffing, long working hours and poor communication structures between professionals. This case has also highlighted the detrimental effect of the 'blame culture'. There is a lot to be learnt from Dr Bawa-Garba, who throughout her journey has been critically honest of her errors, when she unselfishly stated that she hoped the decision would in 'some way improve working conditions of many junior doctors'. It is this ethos of a learning, not blaming, culture that will ensure the safety of patients, and staff, within the NHS.

Paramedics must uphold the highest standards of clinical care and also record keeping, as required by the Health and Care Professions Council (2014). It is the accurate record of care that will be of most use during an allegation of negligence, which may be several months or years after the initial care episode.

Learning from Error

In 2005 and 2010, the NPSA published *Medical Error*, which are guidance booklets that provide advice and guidance for junior doctors on preventing and reporting patient safety incidents. In both versions, senior doctors discuss mistakes they have made and how they have learnt from them, and the second (2010) version contains key steps for how to report something that does go wrong, including how to handle complaints.

These documents are incredibly important. As well as providing a useful tool for reporting mistakes, they contain stories where mistakes are talked about, the errors made and the lessons learnt. Importantly, these examples come from some of the greatest contemporary clinical leaders in medicine, demonstrating that everyone can make mistakes, but it is how they are learned from that results in the development of a safer and more effective health system, both in the NHS and outside of it. These also align with the Department of Health's vision for a learning, not blaming, culture (2015).

Acknowledging that an error took place requires personal insight, courage and a desire to improve. These are characteristics that are fundamental to the development of individual clinicians within the healthcare setting and that must be supported by the workforce culture overall. The Health and Care Professions Council places much emphasis on the need for honesty amongst its registrants, and a statutory Duty of Candour (a professional responsibility to be honest with patients when things go wrong) applies to all care providers registered with the Care Quality Commission (CQC). The intention of this regulation is to ensure that providers are open and transparent with service users and others acting lawfully on their behalf in relation to care and treatment. It also sets out specific requirements for providers to follow when things go wrong with care and treatment, including informing people about the incident, providing support, providing honest information and an apology.

Summary

This chapter has considered the legal aspects that make up a clinical negligence claim, paying particular attention to the duty of care and causation. What we present here is an introduction to these concepts, and we would recommend those who are looking for a more comprehensive understanding to read *Medical Law and Ethics* by Jonathan Herring. We also discuss the problems with the current system and how the healthcare culture may learn from error. The current system does not yet encourage an open culture whereby health professionals can openly learn from their mistakes, but the law does ensure that those who behaved wrongly can be held to account. Whilst more needs to be done to develop the culture of transparency within the health service, individual clinicians must be willing to create change by talking openly and honestly about mistakes they may make, demonstrate they have learned from them and encourage others to learn from them too. This process of learning not only creates a transparent culture, but also creates a learning environment and ultimately a safer environment for patient care.

Recommended Reading

Cohen, D (2017) Back to blame: the Bawa-Garba case and the patient safety agenda. *BMJ*, 359(j5534). doi: https://doi.org/10.1136/bmj.j5534.

Herring, J (2016) *Medical Law and Ethics*, 6th ed. Oxford: Oxford University Press.

Johannsson, H and Rook, W (2018) Avoiding blame and liability is vital to learning from errors and engineering a safer NHS. *BMJ*, 360(k447). doi: https://doi.org/10.1136/bmj.k447.

National Patient Safety Agency (2005) *Medical Error.* Available at: www.nrls.npsa.nhs.uk/resources/?EntryId45=61579.

References

Bristol Royal Infirmary Inquiry (2001) *Learning from Bristol: The Report of the Public Inquiry into children's heart surgery at the Bristol Royal Infirmary 1984–1995*. Available at: http://webarchive.nationalarchives.gov.uk/20090811143822/http://www.bristol-inquiry.org.uk/final_report/the_report.pdf.

Cohen, D (2017) Back to blame: the Bawa-Garba case and the patient safety agenda. *BMJ*, 359(j5534). doi: https://doi.org/10.1136/bmj.j5534.

Department of Health (2001) *An Organisation with a Memory: Report of an Expert Group on Learning from Adverse Events in the NHS Chaired by the Chief Medical Officer*. Available at: www.aagbi.org/sites/default/files/An%20organisation%20with%20a%20memory.pdf.

Department of Health (2015) *Learning Not Blaming*. Available at: https://assets.publishing.service.gov.uk/government/uploads/system/uploads/attachment_data/file/445640/Learning_not_blaming_acc.pdf.

Department of Health (2017) *Introducing Fixed Recoverable Costs in Lower Value Clinical Negligence Claims: A Consultation*. Available at: www.gov.uk/government/uploads/system/uploads/attachment_data/file/586641/FRC_consultation.pdf.

Douglas, T (2009) Medical injury compensation: beyond 'no-fault'. *Medical Law Review*, 17(1). doi: https://doi.org/10.1093/medlaw/fwn022.

Dyer, C (2015) Paediatrician found guilty of manslaughter after boy's death from septic shock. *BMJ*, 351:h5969. doi: https://doi.org/10.1136/bmj.h5969.

Dyer, C (2017) Doctor convicted of manslaughter is suspended from register for a year. *BMJ*, 357:j2928. doi: https://doi.org/10.1136/bmj.j2928.

Health and Care Professions Council (2014) Standards of Proficiency – Paramedics. London: HCPC.

Johannsson, H and Rook, W (2018) Avoiding blame and liability is vital to learning from errors and engineering a safer NHS. *BMJ*, 360(k447). doi: https://doi.org/10.1136/bmj.k447.

Mulheron, R (2010) Trumping *Bolam*: a critical legal analysis of *Bolitho*'s 'gloss. *Cambridge Law Journal*, 69(3): 609–38.

NHS England (2015) *Serious Incident Framework*. Available at: https://www.england.nhs.uk/wp-content/uploads/2015/04/serious-incidnt-framwrk-upd.pdf.

NHS Improvement (2016) *Patient safety incident reporting and responding to Patient Safety Alerts*. Available at: https://improvement.nhs.uk/news-alerts/patient-safety-incident-reporting-and-responding-patient-safety-alerts.

NHS Resolution (2017a) *Annual Report and Accounts 2016/17*. Available at: https://resolution.nhs.uk/wp-content/uploads/2017/07/NHS-Resolution-Annual-report-and-accounts-2016_17.pdf.

NHS Resolution (2017b) *Delivering Fair Resolution and Learning from Harm: Our Strategy to 2022*. Available at: https://resolution.nhs.uk/wp-content/uploads/2017/04/NHS-Resolution-Our-strategy-to-2022-1.pdf.

Samanta, J and Samanta, A (2014) *Concentrate Medical Law*. Oxford: Oxford University Press.

The Stationery Office (2013) *Report of the Mid Staffordshire NHS Foundation Trust Public Inquiry: Executive Summary*. London: The Stationery Office.

Wallis, KA (2017) No-fault, no difference: no-fault compensation for medical injury and healthcare ethics and practice. *British Journal of General Practice*, 67(654). doi: https://doi.org/10.3399/bjgp17X688777.

UK Cases

Antoniades v East Sussex Hospitals NHS Trust [2007] EWHC 517 (QB)

Barnett v Chelsea and Kensington Hospital Management Committee [1969] 2 WLR 42

Bolam v Friern Hospital Management Committee [1957] 1 WLR 582

Bolitho v Hackney Health Authority [1997] 1 All ER 771

Border v Lewisham and Greenwich NHS Trust [2015] EWCA Civ 8

Burne v A [2006] EWCA Civ 24

C v North Cumbria University Hospitals NHS Trust [2014] EWHC 61 (QB)

De Freitas v O'Brien [1995] 6 Med LR 108

Donoghue v Stevenson [1932] UKHL 100

General Medical Council v Bawa-Garba [2018] EWHC 76

Hanson v Airedale Hospital NHS Trust [2003] CLY 2989 (QB)

Hayes v South East Coast Ambulance Service [2015] EWHC 18 (QB)

Horton v Evans [2006] EWHC 2808 (QB)

Jones v Manchester Corporation [1952] 2 QB 852

Judge v Huntingdon Health Authority [1995] 6 Med LR 223

Kent v Griffiths [2000] 2 ER 474

Marriott v West Midlands Health Authority [1999] LI Med Rep 23

Maynard v West Midlands Regional Health Authority [1985] 1 All ER 635

Montgomery v Lanarkshire Health Board [2015] SC 11 [2015] 1 AC 1430

Mulholland v Medway NHS Foundation Trust [2015] EWHC 268 (QB)

Richards v Swansea NHS Trust [2007] EWHC 487 (QB)

R v Adomako [1995] AC 171

Smith v Southampton University Hospital NHS Trust [2007] EXCA Civ 387

Stockdale v Nicholls [1993] 4 Med LR 190

Wilsher v Essex Area Health Authority [1986] AC 1074

Chapter 9

Legislation Relating to Mental Health

Samantha McCabe-Hogan

Introduction

Mental health is a complex condition that has many facets and can be considered a time-consuming affair in practice for paramedics. This chapter is designed to provide some insight into the different legislations concerning mental health across the UK, starting with the history of legislation concerning the current Mental Health Act 1983 and how the UK developed government policies to protect patients and the general public.

The World Health Organization (WHO) (2014) defines mental health as:

A state of wellbeing in which every individual realises his or her own potential, can cope with the normal stresses of life, can work productively and fruitfully, and is able to contribute to his or her community.

This, then, implies a myriad of causes to mental ill health, such as lifestyle choices, the environment and the self-realisation of the individual. However:

Mental ill health, like physical ill health, often has its roots in the interaction between the individual's genetic, biological, neurodevelopmental and other fundamental attributes. Like so many healthcare conditions, it is the complex interaction between the individual and the environment in which she or he grows up, works in, lives in, that can protect against, or trigger, the development of mental illness (Strathdee 2015).

Whilst these statistics provide some insight, it is important that paramedics have a good understanding of mental health issues which they may encounter in clinical practice. The quality of clinical care can have important effects on patients' subsequent engagement with health and care services, and may also have an impact on long-term outcomes.

> **Pause for Thought**
>
> Statistics concerning the problems associated with mental health are alarming:
> - At least one in four people will experience a mental health problem at some point in their life and one in six adults has a mental health problem at any one time (Department of Health 2011, p. 8).
> - Almost half of all adults will experience at least one episode of depression during their lifetime (Department of Health 2011, p. 8).
> - Evidence suggests that 12.7% of all sickness absence days in the UK can be attributed to mental health conditions (Office for National Statistics 2014).
> - In England, one in six people report experiencing a common mental health problem (such as anxiety and depression) in any given week (McManus et al. 2016).
> - 75% of young people with a mental health problem are not receiving treatment (Children's Commissioner for England 2016).

Mental health legislation provides legal protection for people with mental ill health. Under common law, a competent patient may refuse treatment if they wish, even if it is against what is considered by another to be in their best interests. A patient may be given treatment without their consent if they are not competent to make the decision themselves, for example, if they are unconscious or in cardiac arrest. However, this tends to be done under the assumption that treatment will either result in competence and will allow the patient to then make further decisions, or the patient will remain incompetent but will not resist treatment. In the case of mental ill health, patients may require treatment, but be incompetent and resistant to treatment for some time. In such cases, the common law is not adequate to either detain or protect patients. There have been high-profile cases in the last 20 years that have challenged government policy on the management of mental ill health, such as the case of Michael Stone (to devastating effect). We will discuss his case later on in this chapter.

A Short History of Mental Health Legislation

It is important to understand how mental health legislation has developed over the last few hundred years. During the Middle Ages, it was the community that took care of those perceived to be mentally ill. Care took place in asylums, spread throughout the nation, but perhaps the most famous being London's Bethlem asylum. Founded in 1247, it was known locally as 'Bedlam'; thus, this term became synonymous with chaos, confusion, and poor treatment. It is (sadly) this attitude that has been prevalent until modern times (Kelly, 2017).

Between the late thirteenth century and the sixteenth century in England, when Henry VIII established the Court of Wards and Liveries, the English royal courts oversaw hundreds of inquisitions involving individuals thought to be idiots or 'natural fools' (Buhrer 2014). Their role was to determine through questions whether the 'idiot' could manage their affairs and whether they lacked common sense from birth. If they were found to be an 'idiot', then the Crown seized their property and sold their wardships. Often the people who had suggested that the person was an 'idiot' would be made their guardian and have control over their affairs, although this was sometimes overturned (Buhrer 2014). However, Neugebauer (1978) investigated these documents and found English legal records from the thirteenth century through to the seventeenth century which suggested a very different picture. Neugebauer found that royal officials would investigate alleged 'disturbed' persons and would measure their mental status using a common-sense criterion. Once a person was found to be 'disturbed', guardians would be appointed for their care and protection. Although slightly different, both viewpoints demonstrate that it is likely that the questioning of the accused was not always appropriate.

The eighteenth century also saw a series of Vagrancy Acts that allowed 'lunatics' or 'mad persons' to be detained. However, it was the Lunacy Act of 1890 that first provided safeguards against inappropriate detention, although it did not allow for voluntary admissions. This Act came about due to pressure from the public and their concern for wrongful confinement. There were a plethora of documented cases of wrongful confinement, so the major change from the previous policy was to include a third person who was used to agree the confinement of the person. The new law stipulated that a justice of the peace would appoint a magistrate or county court judge who would have jurisdiction over the issue of legal certification (Takabayashi 2017).

It was the Mental Treatment Act 1930 that began the process that we use today. The Act also allowed for voluntary admissions, a feature that was retained by the Mental Health Act 1959, which stated patients should be admitted informally wherever possible. The Mental Health Act 1983 provided legislation for England and Wales on the reception, care and treatment of patients, as well as the management of their property and other related matters. It allowed for the use of 'sections' to admit patients for treatment against their will, and also informed patients and relatives of their rights if they are subject to this Act.

The Mental Health Act 1983 for England and Wales

The Mental Health Act 2007 amended the categories of disorder in the Mental Health Act 1983 to one single definition of mental disorder. This is a broad definition that does not require a formal diagnosis of any kind – for example, schizophrenia is equal to depression. The emphasis of the Mental Health Act 1983 was on the rights of patients, whereas the 2007 amendments concentrated on the public protection and risk management. However, learning disabilities, alcohol and drug dependence are not covered by this Act. Learning disabilities are not considered a disorder under the current Mental Health Act 1983 and people with a learning disability may not be detained under this Act unless they show 'abnormally aggressive irresponsible behaviour'. Alcohol or drug dependence is also not covered as it is not considered a mental disorder.

Anyone may be subject to the Mental Health Act 1983 if they meet the correct criteria. The two principal criteria are having a known mental health disorder or being thought to have an undiagnosed mental health disorder. It should be borne in mind that meeting these criteria does not necessarily mean that someone would be subject to the Act, only that they *could* be.

In order for someone to be subject to the Mental Health Act 1983, appropriate treatment must be available. Appropriate treatment is defined as medical treatment that is appropriate to the person experiencing mental disorder. Therefore, only those with diagnosed mental health disorders and available treatment could be placed under a section, as defined within the Mental Health Act 1983. This strict guidance has generated a number of complex situations, including the cases of Kerrie Wooltorton and Michael Stone. The impact of these cases has led to the changes in standard treatment provided today. Treatment today will range from counselling services (such as talking therapies) to nursing, psychological interventions, and specialist mental health habitation, rehabilitation and care (Care Quality Commission 2018).

Professional Roles

Part 1, Chapter 2 of the Mental Health Act 1983 deals with professionals approved to section persons under the Mental Health Act 1983.

Doctors

Medically trained doctors who have been approved under Section 12(2) of the Mental Health Act 1983. They would have special experience in the diagnosis and treatment of mental disorders. They are usually consultant psychiatrists or GPs who have a special interest in mental health.

Approved Mental Health Professionals (AMHPs)

These are mental health professionals who have undertaken specialist training in the Mental Health Act 1983. Under the Mental Health Act 1983, this could only be done by approved social workers; however, this now includes any suitable professional, such as psychiatric nurses, clinical psychologists or occupational therapists, as well as social workers.

Approved Clinicians

An approved clinician is a mental health professional who can take responsibility for the treatment of people detained under the Mental Health Act 1983. It is usually a consultant psychiatrist; however, it can be other clinicians who have undertaken specialist training, such as nurses or clinical psychologists.

Responsible Clinicians

When an approved clinician takes responsibility for a specific patient, they become known as the responsible clinician.

Nearest Relatives

The nearest relative has an important role under the Mental Health Act 1983 as they can apply for a person to be detained under a Section 2 or 3 of the Act or to be admitted under guardianship. They can also veto any admission under a Section 3 or guardianship and apply for a person to be discharged from a Section 2 or 3 and from guardianship. A nearest relative is defined by law and as such cannot be chosen. The order of priority is as follows:

- husband/wife/civil partner
- child
- parent
- brother/sister
- grandparent.

Where there is more than one person at a given level, such as more than one child, the eldest takes priority.

Hospital Managers

These are volunteers who are trained in mental health law and who represent the management of the hospital in which a patient is detained. They may be anyone 'authorised by the board of the trust in that behalf' and are usually non-executive directors of the hospital. They have a role in hearing appeals against detention under the Mental Health Act 1983.

Mental Health Review Tribunals

These are specialist panels appointed by the Lord Chancellor and are made up of a doctor, a lawyer and a layperson. They have the power to revoke a section under the Mental Health Act 1983 if the appropriate conditions are not met.

Others

A number of others have limited powers under the Mental Health Act 1983 and include non-approved doctors, registered mental health nurses and police officers.

Mental Health Act Sections for Persons with Mental Disorders

Section 2

Section 2 of the Mental Health Act 1983 is used for admission for assessment and is one of the most commonly used sections. Under Section 2, a person may be held for up to 28 days so that their mental health problems can be assessed. In order for someone to be detained under Section 2, two doctors and an AMHP are required. At least one of the doctors must be approved under Section 12(2) of the Mental Health Act 1983 and the other must either know the person in question or be an approved doctor. If a Section 12(2) approved doctor cannot be found, then two non-approved doctors can apply for the section as an emergency measure.

Detention under Section 2 occurs when examination confirms:

(a) the patient is suffering from 'a mental disorder of a nature or degree that warrants detention in hospital for assessment' (or assessment followed by medical treatment) for at least a limited period; and

(b) the patient ought to be detained in the interests of your own health or safety, or with a view to the protection of others.

People with a learning disability can also be detained under Section 2, but they do not have to exhibit 'abnormally aggressive or seriously irresponsible conduct', which is required for Section 3(37) (as below).

Section 3

Section 3 of the Mental Health Act 1983 allows for admission for treatment of mental disorder and can last up to six months. As with Section 2, two doctors and an AMHP are required to detain someone under Section 3. At least one of the doctors must be approved under Section 12(2) of the Mental Health Act 1983 and the other must either know the person in question or be an approved doctor. If a Section 12(2) approved doctor cannot be found, then two non-approved doctors can apply for the section in an emergency.

Detention under Section 3 occurs when examination confirms:

(a) the patient is suffering from a 'mental disorder of a nature or degree' that makes it appropriate to receive medical treatment in hospital; and

(b) it is necessary for the safety of the patient, or for the protection of others, that such treatment is received, and it cannot be provided unless they are detained under this section and appropriate medical treatment is available.

People with a learning disability can also be detained under Section 3(37), but only if (alongside the above criteria) the person exhibits 'abnormally aggressive or seriously irresponsible conduct'.

Section 4

This is used to admit someone for assessment in situations where a second doctor is unavailable and, as such, a Section 2 cannot be used. It requires an AMHP and a doctor who does not need to be approved. This section lasts for up to 72 hours, during which time a second doctor should attend. If the section is to be upheld, then it should be converted to a Section 2.

Section 135

This section is applied for by a magistrate for one of two purposes. The first is as a warrant to gain access to someone in order to assess their mental state. The second is to take or retake a person who is liable to be detained under the Mental Health Act 1983. This section allows any police constable to either enter premises to gain access to someone and/or to remove that person to a place of safety.

In paramedic practice, the use of Section 135 would mean that if the paramedic was unable to gain access to a person who may have an established mental health disorder or may need to be assessed for a mental health disorder, the police need to be requested for support in order to gain access. However, if a warrant has not been approved, then a paramedic may need to initiate a magistrate's order to gain access to the property and the patient. Since this is a lengthy process, the provision under Section 135 is not often used in paramedic practice, although it remains an option that clinicians should be aware of if they encounter a situation that may require the authority of Section 135.

Section 136

This is perhaps the section that is most frequently encountered by frontline ambulance staff. It applies to mentally disordered persons in public places and allows a police constable to remove that person to a place of safety so that they can be examined by an approved doctor and/or an AMHP. It is important to clarify that Section 136 is for use by a police constable, not by a paramedic, and whilst this can only apply to persons in the public, if a person was in a public place and has subsequently entered a private dwelling, they may still be subject to the authority provided for by Section 136.

A Place of Safety

On 11 December 2017, changes to Sections 136 (1c)(d) and 136A(2)(3) of the Mental Health Act 1983 came into force and are outlined in the Mental Health Act 1983 (Places of Safety) Regulations 2017:

1. *A police station is no longer a place of safety, unless the below criteria can be met.*

    (i) *the behaviour of A poses an imminent risk of serious injury or death to A, or to another person,*

    (ii) *because of that risk, no place of safety other than a police station in the relevant police area can reasonably be expected to detain A, and*

    (iii) *the requirement in sub-paragraph (b) of regulation 4(1) will be met, and where the decision-maker is not an officer of the rank of inspector or above, an officer of that rank or above authorises that A may be removed to, kept at, or taken to a place of safety that is a police station.*

2. *Before determining that the circumstances in paragraphs (i) to (iii) of paragraph (1) (a) exist, a decision-maker who is a constable must, if it is reasonably practicable to do so, consult—*

    (a) *a registered medical practitioner,*

    (b) *a registered nurse,*

    (c) *an approved mental health professional, or*

    (d) *a person of a description specified in regulation 8(1).*

This means that in most circumstances, a police station is not a place of safety and must only be used as a last resort. If a police officer is considering using a police station, they must consult with a healthcare professional. Whilst this would (and should) usually be a professional with specific mental health competency, it could be a paramedic (Regulation 2). Importantly, under the 2017 amendments, a police station is no longer a legal place of safety for any child. The decision to use a police station as a place of safety for an adult must be authorised by an officer of the rank of inspector or above.

Treatment under the Mental Health Act 1983

Community Treatment under the Mental Health Act 1983

Under the Mental Health Act 1983, there are three principal routes to gain community treatment:

- guardianship
- Section 17 leave
- Supervised Community Treatment Orders.

Guardianship

This is applied for by local authorities for persons over the age of 16. The person needs to be diagnosed with a mental disorder and it needs to be in the person's best interests.

Section 17 Leave

This section allows the responsible clinician to grant leave from hospital to people otherwise detained under the Mental Health Act 1983. It applies to people already admitted to hospital under Section 2, 3 or 4 of the Mental Health Act 1983.

Supervised Community Treatment Orders

Community Treatment Orders are applied to those patients who are liable for treatment under Sections 3 and 37 (similar to Section 3 but applied to mentally disordered offenders) of the Mental Health Act 1983 and allows for treatment to be given within the community. This treatment cannot be enforced, but the patient may be detained in hospital if the treatment regimen is not followed.

Informal Admission

Despite the many powers that can be enacted under the Mental Health Act 1983, the majority of patients admitted to hospital as a result of mental health problems are done so informally. Formal detention under the Mental Health Act 1983 should be used as a last resort when other options have been attempted or are not considered to be feasible.

The Mental Health (Northern Ireland) Order 1986

The Mental Health (Northern Ireland) 1986 Order is similar to the Mental Health Act 1983; however, there are some difference, alongside a guideline for implementation, that are worth noting.

The Mental Health (Northern Ireland) 1986 Order states that a person may be detained in hospital for assessment of their mental disorder if an application, founded on a medical recommendation, has been made. The application can only be made if the person meets the criteria for admission set out in the Order and if there is no alternative to detention in hospital. Anyone, regardless of age, can be admitted to hospital under the Order if they meet the criteria set out in the Order (Guidelines and Audit Implementation Network 2011).

Non-residents in Northern Ireland (such as refugees, migrant workers, tourists and those who may be considered illegal immigrants) can all be admitted to hospital for assessment and treatment if the criteria under the Order have been met. The Order allows anyone who is not a resident of Northern Ireland to receive assessment and treatment in hospital or care under guardianship.

The criteria for admission looks at whether the person experiencing mental ill health is of a nature which warrants their detention in hospital for assessment and whether failure to detain them would increase the likelihood of serious physical harm to themselves or others. The Order is similar to the Mental Health Act 1983 in that no persons can be detained because of their sexual deviancy, dependency on drugs and alcohol, or personality disorders.

The Mental Health (Scotland) Act 2015

The Mental Health (Scotland) Act 2015 looks to improve mental health services across Scotland and ultimately ensure that people affected by mental ill health are able to access effective treatments in a timely manner. The Act has three main parts:

- *Part 1* outlines the key provisions in the Act, which include: emergency and short-term detention in hospital; the appointment of a named person; outlining of independent advocacy services; safeguarding the patient's interests; and the cross-border transfer of patients outside Scotland and the EU.

- *Part 2* deals explicitly with mental health in criminal cases and how offenders with mental health issues are represented under the Criminal Procedure (Scotland) Act 1995. This includes amended assessment and treatment timescales, and the right to information sharing, and provides variation on certain orders relating to criminal cases.

- *Part 3* focuses on the rights of the victim, including their right to information and the interaction with the Criminal Justice (Scotland) Act 2003. This also allowed the creation of a Victim Notification Scheme for victims of mentally disordered offenders.

The Mental Health (Wales) Measure 2010

Within Wales, this law places legal duties on local health boards and local authorities about the assessment and treatment of those with mental health problems. It has the overriding aim of helping those with mental health issues by increasing independent mental health advocacy and ensuring care across Wales for all mental health needs.

The Measure has four main parts:

- *Part 1* aims to ensure that more mental health services are available within primary care. It aims to provide a service delivered within and alongside primary care settings, focusing on:

- assessment

- short-term interventions

- information, advice and, where appropriate

- onward referral to other services.

- *Part 2* makes sure that all patients in secondary services have a Care and Treatment (CAT) plan. Care co-ordinators are appointed to guarantee that CAT plans are informed by the service user and their carers/families. This ensures that plans are individually tailored and helps mental health services to focus on the recovery model of care and treatment.

- *Part 3* enables eligible adults discharged from secondary services to refer themselves back to those services if they feel their mental health is becoming worse. This means that service users known to the services can bypass primary care.

- *Part 4* supports every in-patient to have help from an independent mental health advocate, as required and if wanted. This extends the Independent Mental Health Advocacy scheme. It covers patients subject to compulsion under the Mental Health Act 1983 and those in hospital voluntarily.

The Human Rights Act 1998

There are 3 Articles in the Human Rights Act 1998 that are important for mental health and provide the legislation to make sure that all those subject to the Mental Health Act 1983 are supported and not subject to unnecessary treatment or detention.

Article 2: Right to Life

The right to life fundamentally deals with the government taking appropriate measures to safeguard human life by making protection laws. This is why the Mental Health Act 1983 has protection for all persons and includes the protection of the public from some people experiencing mental ill health.

Article 3: Freedom from Torture and Inhuman or Degrading Treatment

Freedom from torture and inhuman or degrading treatment is important for those experiencing mental ill health, as it means that the treatment or detention must not be inhuman and must be appropriate and for the least amount of time.

Article 5: Right to Liberty and Security

This focuses on the individual's freedom from detention and can be linked to Articles 3 of the Human Rights Act 1998. For the Mental Health Act 1983, it is to protect the person from unnecessary detention and to ensure they are not detained for longer than is required.

Each Article has an impact on the autonomy of an individual. The Articles allow persons to accept and decline all healthcare treatment both medically and mentally, whilst allowing persons to be fully informed of any and all treatment options. So, the Mental Health Act 1983 has to take these Articles into account. Although the Mental Health Act 1983 allows persons to be detained, voluntary admission is preferred, and any sectioning of persons is done so as a last result. The Human Rights Act 1998 determines that persons must have autonomy over their life; therefore, the Mental Health Act 1983 must work within this Act and the removal of a person's autonomy must not be done lightly or for any unnecessary length of time.

 Case Studies

There are two famous cases that have encouraged changes in the Mental Health Act 1983 to allow persons to be detained.

Michael Stone

The case of Michael Stone saw amendments made to the Mental Health Act 1983 in 2007 to include protection of the general public. Michael Stone was convicted in 1998 of the murders of Lin and Megan Russell, and the attempted murder of Josie Russell. This case is of interest with regard to mental health as at the time only persons who could be treated could be held under the Mental Health Act 1983.

On 9 July 1996, Lin Russell and her two daughters (Megan and Josie) were walking down a Kent country lane when they were viciously attacked. Lin and Megan were killed, and Josie was severely injured. Over a year later, Michael Stone was arrested and charged with their murders. During the trial, it was discovered that he suffered from mental ill health and an inquiry was set up after the trial to investigate the treatment, care, supervision and services provided to him between 1992 and 1997. He had been in and out of trouble for most of his life, he had previously been treated under section and he had also served a number of prison sentences.

Michael Stone was one of a group of patients who were the most difficult and challenging for the health, social and probation services to deal with at the time. He presented with a combination of problems: a severe antisocial personality disorder, multiple drug and alcohol abuse, and occasionally psychotic symptoms consistent with the adverse effects of drug misuse and/or aspects of his personality disorder. This complex and shifting picture made consistent and accurate diagnosis difficult and untreatable, so he could not be sectioned under the Mental Health Act 1983 at that time (South East Coast Strategic Health

(continued)

Authority 2006). During that period of time, he had been in contact regularly with different services, including psychiatric services, probationary centres and hospitals. In 1994, he was convicted of burglary and unlawful possession of a gun, and was committed to a mental health unit under Section 3. On his discharge and before the murders, he was in contact with the probationary office, social services and mental health services. He had expressed on several occasions allegedly having homicidal thoughts and even stated he wanted to kill children.

At the time of his conviction, there were many conflicting official statements regarding whether Michael was declined voluntary admission and treatment. A statement from social services and the probation office which had been subject to an amendment by the Department of Health stated that Michael was not mentally ill and that he was responsible for his own actions (Francis 2007). Jack Straw, the then Home Secretary, stated that the psychiatric services were responsible for not detaining those persons who were 'untreatable'. However, the Mental Health Act 1983 was clear – unless the mental disorder could be treated, then such individuals could not be sectioned. There were some queries regarding whether the delay in a drug being given to Michael and the increased aggression experienced would have led him to be sectioned. In 2007, the government amended the Mental Health Act 1983, after many debates and defeats of the proposed bill. The changes to the Act meant that persons with personality disorders could be offered 'talking therapy' and therefore could be sectioned for treatment. There were also changes made to the Criminal Justice Act 2003.

Kerrie Wooltorton

Kerrie Wooltorton completed suicide on 19 September 2007 from ethylene glycol toxicity. On admission to hospital, it was discovered that she had consumed 350 ml of antifreeze. However, she did not allow any medical intervention and only wished to be kept 'comfortable'. On admission (via ambulance), she was also in possession of a letter written by her and dated 14 September 2007. This letter was treated as an advance directive.

To whom this may concern, if I come into hospital regarding taking an overdose or any attempt on my life, I would like for NO lifesaving treatment to be given. I would appreciate if you could continue to give medicines to help relieve my discomfort, pain killers, oxygen etc. I would hope these wishes will be carried out without loads if [sic] questioning.

Please be assured that I am 100% aware of the consequences of this and the probable outcome of drinking antifreeze e.g. death in 95–99% of cases and if I survive then kidney failure, I understand and accept them and will take 100% responsibility for this decision.

I am aware that you may think that because I call an ambulance, I therefore want treatment. THIS IS NOT THE CASE! I do however want to be comfortable as nobody wants to die alone and scared and without going into details there are loads of reasons I do not want to die at home which I realise that you will not understand, and I apologise for this.

Please understand that I definitely don't want any form of ventilation, resuscitation or dialysis, these are my wishes, please respect and carry them out.

Kerrie had a history of self-harm and had previously attempted suicide nine times using the same method, but on each of the occasions she had agreed to treatment for the attempt. She died three days after her admission. She did not disclose why this time was different, but it may have been due to genealogical issues.

The doctors treating Kerrie sought advice from several avenues, including legal advice (Szawarski 2013). They decided that as Kerrie had capacity, she had the right to decline treatment. When asked, the doctor in charge of Kerrie's care stated that he knew he was breaking the law if he were to treat Kerrie and that whilst the chance of litigation wasn't on his mind, he was aware that if he had treated Kerrie and she had survived, she would have probably sued (Gabbatt 2009).

Kerrie had a diagnosis of an unstable personality disorder that was untreatable. The coroner, William Armstrong, pronounced the following:

> *Kerrie Anne Wooltorton died as the result of deliberately consuming a poisonous substance in the full knowledge that death could result. She had the capacity to consent to treatment which, it is more likely than not, would have prevented her death. She refused such treatment in full knowledge of the consequences and died as a result.*

This case is important as it requires understanding of the Human Rights Act 1998, the Mental Health Act 1983, the Mental Capacity Act 2005 and advance decisions.

At the time of her death, the Mental Capacity Act 2005 had only been in law for five months. Although the 2007 amendments to the Mental Health Act 1983 had been published, they were not yet law; therefore, as Kerrie had an untreatable mental disorder, she could not be sectioned, although it may be considered that she was possibly suffering from depression, which meant she could have been sectioned. There has been some debate as to whether it was the mental capacity or the advance directive that led to the decision to allow Kerrie to complete her suicide (Muzaffar 2010; Callaghan and Ryan 2011; Szawarski 2013).

The Human Rights Act 1998 was very clear – a person has the right to decide what happens to their own body – and the Mental Capacity Act 2005 states that it should be assumed that someone has capacity unless it can be proven that they lack capacity. The advance directive Kerrie wrote only gave the doctors information that this was not a spur of the moment decision, that this decision had not been taken lightly and that she understood the consequences of her actions.

Muzaffar (2010) suggests that the English courts had considered the validity of an advance decision for the first time in *Re C* (1994), where a sectioned patient refused to have his gangrenous foot removed and was successful in his injunction. Muzaffar goes on to say that this ruling made a capacitous advance refusal of treatment binding and that there was no requirement for formal

(continued)

documentation. However, until her death, it was documented that Kerrie never lost her mental capacity, therefore an advance decision was never in use.

This case has led to several articles and many authors debating the decisions made by the doctors and the subsequent coroner's report. Many pose good questions as to why Kerrie was not sectioned as she had been previously or why the hospital spoke to everyone except the psychiatrist treating Kerrie. However, the most prevalent question is what changed in Kerrie's life to cause her to make the decision this time to refuse treatment?

Summary

This chapter has covered mental health legislation in relation to the UK. Understanding the development of current legislation from the history of mental health treatment aids us in our understanding of the development of the law today, and in reducing the stigma associated with mental ill health. Laws specific to England, Wales, Scotland and Northern Ireland have been outlined clearly. Unlike other chapters within this book, the two case studies are based on real examples from clinical practice, examples which led to changes in legislation.

Recommended Reading

Barcham, C (2012). *The Pocketbook Guide to Mental Health Act Assessments*, 2nd ed. Maidenhead: Open University Press.

Roberts, M (2018). *Understanding Mental Health Care*. London: Sage.

References

Bracchi, P (2009) Special investigation: what kind of country have we become if doctors and lawyers allow a disturbed young woman to die? Daily Mail, 10 October. Available at: www .dailymail.co.uk/news/article-1219389/SPECIAL-INVESTIGATION-What-kind-countrydoctors-lawyers-allow-disturbed-young-woman-die.html.

Buhrer, E (2014) Law and mental competency in late medieval England. *Reading Medieval Studies*, 40. Available at: www.medievalists.net/2017/10/law-mental-competency-late-medieval-england.

Callaghan, S and Ryan, C (2011). Refusing medical treatment after attempted suicide: rethinking capacity and coercive treatment in light of the Kerrie Wooltorton case. *Journal of Law Medicine*, 18(4): 811–19.

Care Quality Commission (2018) *Monitoring the Mental Health Act in 2016/17*. Available at: www.cqc .org.uk/publications/major-report/monitoring-mental-health-act-report.

Children's Commissioner for England (2016) *Lightening Review: Access to Child and Adolescent Mental Health Services*. Available at: https://www.childrenscommissioner.gov.uk/wp-content/uploads/2017/06/Childrens-Commissioners-Mental-Health-Lightning-Review.pdf.

Department of Health (2011). *No health without mental health*. London: Her Majesty's Stationery Office.

Francis, R (2007) The Michael Stone Inquiry – A Reflection. *International Journal of Mental Health and Capacity Law*, 15. Available at: www.northumbriajournals.co.uk/index.php/IJMHMCL/article/view/199/194.

Gabbatt, A (2009) Doctors acted legally in 'living will' suicide case. *The Guardian*, 1 October 2009. Available at: www.theguardian.com/society/2009/oct/01/living-will-suicide-legal.

Guidelines and Audit Implementation Network (2011) *Guidelines on the Use of the Mental Health (Northern Ireland) Order 1986*. Available at: www.rqia.org.uk/RQIA/files/4e/4ee9f634-be47-4398-afc9-906a20ff3198.pdf.

Kelly, E (2017) '*Mental Illness During the Middle Ages' Science and its Times: Understanding the Social Significance of Scientific Discovery*. Gale Press: LA.

McLean, S (2009) Sheila McLean on advance directives and the case of Kerrie Wooltorton. Available at: https://blogs.bmj.com/bmj/2009/10/01/sheila-mclean-on-advance-directives-and-the-case-of-kerrie-wooltorton.

McManus, S et al, (eds) (2016 *Mental Health and Wellbeing in England: Adult Psychiatric Morbidity Survey 2014*. Leeds: NHS Digital.

Muzaffar, S (2010) 'To treat or not to treat': Kerrie Wooltorton, lessons to learn. *Emergency Medicine Journal*, 28(9): 741–44.

Neugebauer, R (1978) Treatment of the mentally ill in medieval and early modern England: a reappraisal. *History of Behavioral Sciences*, 14(2): 158–69.

Northern Ireland Commissioner for Children and Young People (2017) *Child and Adolescent Mental Health in NI*. Available at: www.NI.org/media/2810/niccy-scoping-paper-mental-health-review-apr-2017.pdf.

Office for National Statistics (2014) *Full Report: Sickness Absence on the Labour Market, February 2014*. Available at: https://webarchive.nationalarchives.gov.uk/20160105160709/http://www.ons.gov.uk/ons/dcp171776_353899.pdf.

South East Coast Strategic Health Authority (2006) *Report of the Independent Inquiry into the Care and Treatment of Michael Stone*. Available at: http://hundredfamilies.org/wp/wp-content/uploads/2013/12/MICHAEL_STONE_JULY96.pdf.

Strathedee, G (2015) *A defining moment in mental health care*. Available at: www.england.nhs.uk/blog/geraldine-strathdee-8.

Szawarski, P (2013). Classic cases revisited: the suicide of Kerrie Wooltorton. *Journal of Intensive Care Society*, 14(3). Available at: http://journals.sagepub.com/doi/pdf/10.1177/175114371301400307.

Takabayashi, A (2017) Surviving the Lunacy Act of 1890: English psychiatrists and professional development during the early twentieth century. *Medical History*, 61(2): 246–69.

World Health Organization (WHO) (2014) *Mental Health: A State of Well-Being*. Available at: www.who.int/features/factfiles/mental_health/en.

UK Cases

Re C [1994] 1 All ER 819; [1994] 1 WLR 290

UK Legislation

Criminal Justice Act 2003

Criminal Justice (Scotland) Act 2003

Human Rights Act 1998

Lunacy Act of 1890

Mental Capacity Act 2005

Mental Capacity (NI) Act 2016

Mental Health Act 1959

Mental Health Act 1983

Mental Health Act, 2007

Mental Health (Northern Ireland) Order, 1986

Mental Health Act 1983 (Places of Safety) Regulations 2017

Mental Health (Scotland) Act 2015

Mental Health (Wales) Measure 2010

Mental Treatment Act 1930

Vagrancy Act 1824

Chapter 10

Assessing Mental Capacity

Edd Bartlett

Introduction

The Mental Capacity Act 2005 was enacted in 2007 and sets out the legal framework for assessing whether a patient has the capacity to make a specific decision, and making decisions on the behalf of patients found to lack capacity (Office of the Public Guardian 2013). It has a golden thread that there should be an initial presumption of capacity for all those over the age of 16 (Heywood 2014).

In 2015, the House of Lords published its report on whether the Mental Capacity Act 2005 was being utilised as Parliament intended. It found that: 'Capacity assessments are not often carried out [and] when they are, the quality is often poor' (House of Lords 2015, p. 8). Two years on, its concerns about clinicians' understanding and utilisation of the Act are still demonstrated, with concern about capacity assessments and best interests decisions often coming up in Serious Case Reviews and Safeguarding Adults Reviews (Cooper and White 2017). A review of 27 Safeguarding Adult Reviews (SARs) in London found that in 21 of the reviews, capacity assessment and best interests decision making was mentioned, but only positively in one review (Braye and Preston-Shoot 2017).

It is crucial that paramedics are able to competently assess mental capacity and make best interests decisions. Even if a paramedic requires assistance to complete the capacity assessment from a more senior paramedic or another healthcare professional, they cannot delegate responsibility for assessing capacity to that person (39 Essex Chambers 2016, p. 3). If a paramedic does not reasonably believe that on the balance of probabilities a patient lacks capacity and acts in their best interests, they will not have a defence (39 Essex Chambers 2016, p. 3), which could result in them being found guilty of the tort of battery.

Scotland

In Scotland, issues surrounding decision making for patients who lack capacity is detailed within the Adults with Incapacity (Scotland) Act 2000, with the Mental Health (Care and Treatment) (Scotland) Act 2003 providing information about those with mental health problems. The Adults with Incapacity (Scotland) Act 2000 provides the legal framework for decision making with regard to adults who lack capacity in Scotland in relation to welfare, property, financial affairs and medical treatment.

The Adults with Incapacity (Scotland) Act 2000 defines incapacity as occurring when a person is unable to act, make decisions, communicate those decisions, understand decisions and retain memory of those decisions.

Northern Ireland

In Northern Ireland, the Mental Capacity Act (Northern Ireland) 2016 covers the legalities surrounding mental capacity, and making best interests decisions for those who lack capacity. At the time of writing, this Act is still being implemented in Northern Ireland. The Act outlines, in a very similar way to the law in England and Wales, that an individual who is unable to make a decision about their care lacks capacity if they are unable to understand relevant information, are unable to retain the information for the time required to make the decision, are unable to understand the relevance of the information and to use or weigh such information as part of the decision-making process, and are unable to communicate their decision by any means.

The Mental Capacity Act and Autonomy

The right to autonomy is considered a core right in medical ethics and is central to gaining consent for medical treatment. It has long been recognised by medical ethicists that even if a patient is making an unwise decision, this is not in itself a good reason for paternalistic interference (Harris 1985). In order for a clinician to gain real consent from a patient for any treatment or intervention, the patient must be fully informed, free from undue influence and have capacity. If the patient is found to be able to give real consent and they choose not to, this decision must be respected.

Re C (Adult: Refusal of Treatment) (1994)

This case was heard prior to the Mental Capacity Act 2005, so did not follow its legislative framework.

The Decision

Amputation of a gangrenous foot.

The Patient

C was a patient at Broadmoor and suffered from chronic paranoid schizophrenia.

Assessment

C's general capacity was not impaired enough by his illness to prevent him from being able to understand the nature, purpose and effects of the treatment.

C understood that the doctors thought he would die without treatment.

Outcome

C accepted only conservative treatment, from which his foot made a recovery.

The case of *Re C (Adult: Refusal of Treatment)* (1994) set a precedent in common law that a person must not be treated as being unable to make a decision to refuse medical treatment simply because they make an unwise decision. It is the approach used in *Re C* that has influenced the statutory framework for assessing capacity outlined in the Mental Capacity Act 2005.

The patient's right to refuse treatment or not be subjected to excessive force or coercion if they are being treated in their best interests has been given further weight by the Human Rights Act 1998. The Articles in Schedule 1 to the Human Rights Act gives patients the following rights (relevant to healthcare decisions):

Article 3 – The right to not be subjected to torture or inhuman or degrading treatment.
Article 5 – The right to liberty and security of person.
Article 8 – The right to private and family life.
Article 9 – The right to freedom of thought, conscience and religion.

The Article 3 right that prohibits torture or inhuman or degrading treatment is an *absolute* right, which means that it is never acceptable to treat a person to inhuman or degrading treatment, or torture them. *Herczegfalvy v Austria* (1993) is European case law that has influence in the UK. In this case, the European Court of Human Rights found that although the patient had been subject to forced feeding, forced administration of drugs and handcuffed to a bed for more than two weeks, his Article 3 right had not been breached (Hale 2017). This is because there was therapeutic necessity; the threshold for this is high and it is unlikely that medical treatment that is therapeutically necessary would ever be found to be inhuman or degrading treatment (Hale 2017).

The other rights are *qualified* rights, which means that infringement of them is only acceptable in certain circumstances; in the healthcare setting, Article 5 may be enacted for 'the lawful detention of persons for the prevention of the spreading of infectious diseases, of persons of unsound mind, alcoholics or drug addicts or vagrants' (Schedule 1 (Article 5, 1(e)). Articles 8 and 9 may only be infringed if it is deemed to be necessary in certain circumstances set out by the Human Rights Act; these include 'public safety', 'for the protection of health or morals' and 'the protection of the rights and freedom of others' (Schedule 1 (Articles 8–9)).

These rights protect patients from paternalistic interference by healthcare professionals. They apply regardless of whether a patient has or lacks capacity; a patient who lacks capacity is not suddenly stripped of their rights and made subject to paternalistic intervention by clinicians, and it is recognised that it is seldom in the best interests of a patient who lacks capacity to be subjected to forced treatment (Jackson 2016).

Assessing Capacity

When conducting a capacity assessment, the five statutory principles (see below) set out by the Mental Capacity Act should be at the forefront of the minds of those involved. The Act provides a two-stage test to assess if a patient has capacity: a diagnostic and functional test. Both tests must be completed before a conclusion about the patient's capacity to make a specific decision at a specific time can be made on the balance of probabilities (sections 2–3 of the Mental Capacity Act 2005).

The Principles (Section 1 of the Mental Capacity Act 2005)

1. A person must be assumed to have capacity unless it is established that he lacks capacity.

2. A person is not to be treated as unable to make a decision unless all practicable steps to help him to do so have been taken without success.

3. A person is not to be treated as unable to make a decision merely because he makes an unwise decision.

4. An act done, or decision made, under this Act for or on behalf of a person who lacks capacity must be done, or made, in his best interests.

5. Before the act is done, or the decision is made, regard must be had to whether the purpose for which it is needed can be as effectively achieved in a way that is less restrictive of the person's rights and freedom of action.

A capacity assessment should be considered for any patient over the age of 16 who is making a specific decision and meets the diagnostic threshold set by the Act, as determined by the diagnostic test.

Stage 1: The Diagnostic Test (Section 2(1) of the Mental Capacity Act 2005)

For the purposes of this Act, a person lacks capacity in relation to a matter if at the material time he is unable to make a decision for himself in relation to the matter *because of an impairment of, or a disturbance in the functioning of, the mind or brain.*

[Emphasis added]

This is the first stage of the capacity assessment: if the person does not have an impairment of or a disturbance in the functioning of the mind or brain, they cannot be found to lack capacity to make the decision and the capacity assessment ends at the first stage. However, if they are found to be under coercion or undue influence, this could also mean they are unable to make the decision (*Re T (Adult: Refusal of Treatment)* (1993)).

The Mental Capacity Act Code of Practice gives *examples* of what might cause an impairment of the mind or brain, including: dementia, some forms of mental illness, symptoms of alcohol and drug use, significant learning difficulties, concussion and brain damage (Office of the Public Guardian 2013).

If a diagnostic test is required to be undertaken, but the patient is believed to have an impairment of or a disturbance in the functioning of their mind or brain, the assessment progresses to the second stage of the capacity assessment.

Stage 2: The Functional Test (Section 3(1) of the Mental Capacity Act 2005)

[A] person is unable to make a decision for himself if he is unable –

a) to understand the information relevant to the decision,

b) to retain that information,

c) to use or weigh that information as part of the process of making the decision, or

d) to communicate his decision (whether by talking, using sign language *or any other means*). [Emphasis added]

If the patient was to fail the functional test and be found to lack capacity, they must be unable to do one or more of the following:

1. Understand the information they have been given that is relevant to the decision they are making.

2. Retain that information long enough to make a decision.

3. Use or weigh up the information they have been given as part of their coming to their decision.

4. Communicate their decision in any way.

If they are unable to do one or more of the above, then on the balance of probabilities, they will be found to lack capacity to make *that specific decision at that specific time*. It is important to note that the Mental Capacity Act does not ask for a definitive assertion that the patient lacks capacity, but, instead, that the person carrying out the assessment believes that the patient lacks capacity on the balance of probabilities.

Essentially, it should seem more likely that the patient lacks capacity and the clinician should be able to provide reasons for this in the documentation. Good documentation is essential as this is what will be referred to if the capacity assessment is ever called into question.

✸ Case Study: Mrs L

A 999 call comes in at 23:30 for Mrs L, an 86-year-old female who has had a period of unresponsiveness and unilateral weakness. This lasted for about 15 minutes and following the paramedic's arrival, she has returned to her normal self;

(continued)

according to her daughter. Following the paramedic's assessment, it is also noted that Mrs L is hypertensive. Her daughter says that Mrs L is due to have a 'memory assessment'; she thinks this is for concerns that she has some cognitive decline.

The paramedic is concerned that Mrs L is at risk of having a stroke, calculating her $ABCD^2$ score as five (moderate risk). The paramedic advises that it would be a good idea to go to hospital for further assessment and medication review, particularly as Mrs L is already on anticoagulation treatment (National Institute for Health and Care Excellence (NICE) 2017).

Mrs L states that while she appreciates the paramedic's concerns and acknowledges that there would be risks to not being taken to the Emergency Department (ED), she would prefer to stay at home. She is aware that she could have a stroke and that there is a risk of permanent disability; however, she states that she is fed up with hospital and that she doesn't want to go. Instead, she will let her GP know in the morning and they can review her medication; her daughter will stay with her and will call 999 if she has any further symptoms.

Applying the Diagnostic Test to Mrs L

It is important that the paramedic starts from the rebuttable presumption that Mrs L has capacity, so the first test that needs to be applied is the diagnostic test. Does Mrs L have an impairment of or a disturbance in the functioning of the mind or brain? It is important to note that Mrs L has no formal diagnosis of dementia or cognitive impairment; she is only due for an assessment. As such, the paramedic should not jump to any conclusions about her capacity.

The diagnostic test does not require a formal diagnosis to support the decision that the person fails the test, although being able to document a condition such as dementia or a learning disability will make establishing an impairment of or a disturbance in the functioning of the mind or brain easier. *It is crucial that this is not interpreted as meaning that the person cannot make the decision – the second (functional) test must still be performed and documented.*

As Mrs L does not have a formal diagnosis, this means that she fails the diagnostic test. The paramedic must document what leads them to believe that she has an impairment of or a disturbance in the functioning of the mind or brain. In Mrs L's case, this could be that there have been concerns about her cognition and memory, or that she has just had a neurological event. Other things could be the ingestion of alcohol or any other substances that affect cognition, fatigue, pain or trauma (this is not an exhaustive list).

Once the paramedic has found that Mrs L has failed the diagnostic test, they can move on to the functional test. This is the test that establishes whether Mrs L has the capacity to make the specific decision to stay at home and not go to hospital. If Mrs L is found to be unable to do any one of the following – understand, use and weigh, retain or communicate information – she will be found to be unable to make the decision on her own and the paramedic will have to make a decision in her best interests.

Applying the Functional Test to Mrs L

In order to apply the functional test, it is crucial that the paramedic is clear on what decision they are asking Mrs L to make and how significant the decision is. The threshold is higher for decisions that could be life-threatening or life-changing. So, for example, the decision to have sugar in your tea is not as significant as the decision to decline conveyance to hospital when significant changes have been found on your electrocardiogram (ECG). It is also important that the paramedic is able to give the patient sufficient information in order for them to make an informed decision and weigh up that information as part of the decision-making process.

Understand

Mrs L must be able to understand the relevant information as to why the paramedic wants her to go to hospital. The level of understanding does not have to be that of the paramedic or an expert; instead, they should be able to demonstrate a *broad, general understanding of the kind that is expected from the population at large* (*Heart of England NHS Trust v JB* (2014); 39 Essex Chambers 2014).

The Mental Capacity Act Code of Practice advises that relevant information includes:

- the nature of the decision;
- the reason why the decision is needed; and
- the likely effects of deciding one way or another, or making no decision at all.

(Office of the Public Guardian 2013).

In the case of Mrs L, this is a broad understanding of the risk of not going to hospital – that she may have a stroke and that she may suffer permanent disability and premature death as a result of declining conveyance to the ED.

Retain

Mrs L must be able to retain this information for long enough to be able to use and weigh it up. The Act and the Code are very clear that if a person is only able to retain information for a short while, they should not automatically be assumed to lack capacity (Office of the Public Guardian 2013; section 3(3) of the Mental Capacity Act 2005).

Use and Weigh

To demonstrate that she is able to use and weigh the information that Mrs L has understood and is retaining, she must be able to apply it to the decision she is making. *Re MB (Adult: Medical Treatment)* (1997) is a good example of someone being unable to use and weigh up information as part of their decision-making process. MB was due to have an emergency caesarean section, but refused due to extreme needle phobia. The court found that due to her fear and panic, she

(continued)

was unable to use and weigh up the information relating to the risk to her and her baby against her fear of needles, and therefore she temporarily lacked capacity to refuse the caesarean section.

Mrs L is able to demonstrate that she weighed up her previous experiences at hospital with her preference to stay at home. It is essential that she is able to demonstrate that she is weighing up the risks such as significant disability and premature death as part of her decision making; if she is convinced that there is no risk to staying at home, the paramedic should be concerned about her ability to use and weigh up information.

Communicate

Mrs L is able to verbally communicate her decision. It is important that if a person has any barriers to communicating information, they are assisted in communicating their decision. For patients with disabilities, where this means that their ability to communicate information is reduced or restricted to 'yes' or 'no' answers, it may be appropriate to seek assistance from people who know the person well in order to ensure that all practical steps have been taken to help them to communicate their decision (section 1(3) of the Mental Capacity Act 2005).

Best Interests Decisions

Following a capacity assessment, the patient may be found to lack capacity to make the decision. This means that a decision must be made in the patient's best interests, unless the decision can wait until the patient regains capacity (if the impairment of or a disturbance in the functioning of the mind or brain is temporary) (Mental Capacity Act 2005, Explanatory Notes (EN) 29).

This is in accordance with the fourth principle of the Mental Capacity Act 2005: 'an act done, or decision made, under this Act for or on behalf of a person who lacks capacity must be done, or made, in his best interests' (section 1(5) of the Mental Capacity Act 2005). One of the few exceptions to this is where the patient has made an advance decision for the refusal of life-sustaining treatment; this will be covered later in this chapter (Office of the Public Guardian 2013).

The fifth principle of the Mental Capacity Act 2005 must also be followed when making a best interests decision: 'Before the act is done, or the decision is made, regard must be had to whether the purpose for which it is needed can be as effectively achieved in a way that is less restrictive of the person's rights and freedom of action' (section 1(6) of the Mental Capacity Act 2005).

Only if a decision is made that is in the patient's best interests will the paramedic be protected from the tort of battery; however, they are not protected from being found clinically negligent. The Mental Capacity Act offers guidance on how a best interests decision should be made in section 4, with guidance offered within the Code.

A best interests decision *must* be documented and include the following information:

- how the decision about the person's best interests was reached;
- what the reasons for reaching the decision were;
- who was consulted to help work out best interests; and
- what particular factors were taken into account (Office of the Public Guardian 2013).

When making a best interests decision for a person, the paramedic should always have section 4(4), (6) and (7) of the Act in mind.

Best Interests (Section 4(4), (6) and (7) of the Mental Capacity Act 2005)

(4) He must, so far as reasonably practicable, permit and encourage the person to participate, or to improve his ability to participate, as fully as possible in any act done for him and any decision affecting him.

(6) He must consider, so far as is reasonably ascertainable —

a) the person's past and present wishes and feelings (and, in particular, any relevant written statement made by him when he had capacity),

b) the beliefs and values that would be likely to influence his decision if he had capacity, and

c) the other factors that he would be likely to consider if he were able to do so.

(7) He must take into account, if it is practicable and appropriate to consult them, the views of —

a) anyone named by the person as someone to be consulted on the matter in question or on matters of that kind,

b) anyone engaged in caring for the person or interested in his welfare,

c) any donee of a lasting power of attorney granted by the person, and

d) any deputy appointed for the person by the court,

as to what would be in the person's best interests and, in particular, as to the matters mentioned in subsection (6).

The person's past and present wishes and feelings *must* be given significant weight when a best interests decision is being made. These can be established by the assessor by consulting with anyone outlined in section 4(7). There has been a significant move away from a paternalistic approach where best interests decisions are made on the basis of what is considered to be in the patient's *medical* best interests.

Where there is a dispute about a person lacking capacity or whether a treatment is in their best interests, the case will usually be considered by the Court of Protection. The Court of Protection covers:

- the authorisation of deprivation of liberty;
- matters relating to lasting powers of attorney; and
- decisions for people who lack capacity about their welfare or finance.

The extent to which the patient's wishes and feelings are taken into account by the Court of Protection is currently best demonstrated by the case of *Wye Valley NHS Trust v Mr B* (2015).

Wye Valley NHS Trust v Mr B (2015)

The Decision

Amputation of a leg.

The Patient

Mr B had a history of mental illness and type 2 diabetes, which had resulted in a foot ulcer becoming infected. The infection eventually spread to the bone and the hospital considered that amputation of the leg was required to prevent imminent death (39 Essex Chambers 2015).

Assessment

The judge, Peter Jackson J, gave the following rationale for believing on the balance of probabilities that Mr B lacked capacity:

Based on the following evidence, I am satisfied that Mr B does not have the capacity to make treatment decisions about his foot:

1. He suffers from persistent and treatment-resistant Schizoaffective Disorder, otherwise known as Bipolar Affective Disorder with Psychotic Symptoms.

2. In consequence, he experiences auditory hallucinations that tell him whether or not to take his medication: 'If the Lord says it's no, it's no.' Although he did not make a similar connection when speaking about amputation to Dr Glover or to me, he told Ms Chapman that because the Lord doesn't want him to have his leg taken off, he is not doing it.

3. He does not understand the reality of his injury. Asked how things would go if he did not have the operation, he told me that his leg would get better with proper care and if he was allowed to use it.

4. He also mistrusts the doctors to the extent that he expressed the fear that if they put him to sleep for the operation, they could do anything. He did not seem reassured by my telling them that they would not go beyond treatment that the court permitted.

---

5. Whenever anyone speaks to Mr B about treatment for his leg, he becomes agitated and will shut down the conversation so that the pros and cons of the various options cannot be further discussed (para 34).

Best Interests Supporting Information

Peter Jackson J considered Mr B's wishes and feelings to be so significant in his decision making that he went to visit Mr B.

A number of statements that Mr B made strongly influenced Peter Jackson J's decision. These included the following:

I don't want an operation.

I'm not afraid of dying, I know where I'm going. The angels have told me I am going to heaven. I have no regrets. It would be a better life than this.

I don't want to go into a nursing home, [my partner] died there.

I don't want my leg tampered with. I know the seriousness, I just want them to continue what they're doing.

I don't want it. I'm not afraid of death. I don't want interference. Even if I'm going to die, I don't want the operation.

All this was said with great seriousness, and in saying it, Mr B did not appear to be showing florid psychiatric symptoms or to be unduly affected by toxic infection (para 37(1)).

Peter Jackson J also took into consideration the impact that having the operation would have on Mr B's quality of life following the operation and the likelihood that the amputated limb would serve as a constant reminder that his and (Mr B believes) the Lord's wishes had not been respected (para 37(4)).

Best Interests Decision

Peter Jackson J highlighted that the absence of capacity did not mean that Mr B was no longer protected by the European Convention on Human Rights (the Convention) as per the Human Rights Act (1998). In this case, Peter Jackson J considered that Article 2 (the right to life), Article 3 (the right to not be subject to inhuman or degrading treatment) and Article 9 (the right to freedom of religion) were engaged.

It was decided that it was in Mr B's best interests to not receive the treatment. Peter Jackson J concluded:

> I am quite sure that it would not be in Mr B's best interests to take away his little remaining independence and dignity in order to replace it with a future for which he understandably has no appetite and which could only be achieved after a traumatic and uncertain struggle that he and no one else would have to endure. There is a difference between fighting on someone's behalf and just fighting them. Enforcing treatment in this case would surely be the latter (para 45).

Best Interests in Practice

When making a decision in a patient's best interests, the paramedic is protected from being found to have unlawfully touched the patient (the tort of battery) as long as they have met the criteria set out in section 5 of the Mental Capacity Act 2005:

1. Reasonable steps have been taken to establish if the person lacks capacity; and

2. The clinician *reasonably believes* that the person lacks capacity and that the treatment or intervention that they are considering is in the person's best interests.

If restraint is required, a further two criteria must be met (see the section below on restraint and section 6 of the Mental Capacity Act 2005).

So, for example, if the patient lacks capacity and is compliant with treatment being planned (or is unconscious), under section 5 of the Mental Capacity Act 2005, the paramedic is able to treat them in their best interests. See the section on restraint and proportionality below for more details on the situation where the patient lacks capacity and resists treatment.

Best Interests and Life-limiting Conditions

There may be situations where you believe that providing your patient with treatment is not in their best interests. On these occasions, it is important to remember that the starting presumption should always be strongly that it is in the patient's best interests to stay alive (*Aintree University Hospitals NHS Foundation Trust v James* (2014), para 35). As long as the decision-making process set out by the Mental Capacity Act 2005 and demonstrated by the court in *Wye Valley NHS Trust v Mr B* is followed, the decision will be made in the patient's best interests.

It is also important to consider section 4(5) of the Mental Capacity Act 2005: 'Where the determination relates to life-sustaining treatment he must not, in considering whether the treatment is in the best interests of the person concerned, be motivated by a desire to bring about his death.' This section ensures that the Mental Capacity Act cannot be used as a back door to euthanasia.

In practice, paramedics will almost certainly find themselves in a situation where they have a duty of care for a patient who lacks capacity and their holistic best interests do not match what treatment protocols or policies suggest is in the patient's medical best interests, for example, treatment guidance based on national early warning scores.

An example of this would be a patient who is believed to be at the end of their life. A holistic assessment may reveal that interventions to reverse sepsis are unlikely to be effective, the patient may also be frail, and their family may oppose them being acutely admitted to hospital. You could reasonably come to the conclusion that treatment and acute admission are not in the patient's best interests, even though it is likely that sepsis will result in their death.

Any decision like the above is best made as a shared decision and guidance from experts, such as hospice staff, should be sought where possible. It is also important to make sure that contingencies are in place should the patient deteriorate and suffer discomfort or distress. Chapter 12 looks at this in more detail.

Restraint

A patient may be treated in their best interests once the decision has been made that the patient:

1. Has an impairment of, or a disturbance in the functioning of, the mind or brain; and

2. Is unable to do one or more of the following:

   a. Understand the information you have given them

   b. Retain that information for long enough that they can make a decision

   c. Use or weigh the information as part of the decision-making process

   d. Communicate their decision to you by any means; and

3. On the balance of probability lacks capacity; and

4. a. The decision they are making cannot wait until they regain capacity, or

   b. They won't regain capacity without the treatment that they need, or

   c. They won't regain capacity; and

5. The treatment is in their best interests, in line with section 4 of the Act; and

6. There is no valid advance decision to refuse treatment (ADRT) that applies to the treatment you are going to give.

However, the patient may not accept the decision that they need to be treated; in some situations, this may result in them refusing to comply. Such situations are often resolved through good communication and explanation, but sometimes this is not possible or practicable. In such situations, the patient may need to be restrained.

Section 6 of the Mental Capacity Act 2005 outlines when it is acceptable to restrain a person for the purposes of care or treatment. It is very important to recognise that restraint includes both using force and threatening to use force when the person is resisting care or treatment; it also includes restricting the person's liberty of movement, whether or not they resist (section 6(4)). Restraint may only be used if the following four conditions are met:

1. Reasonable steps have been taken to establish if the person lacks capacity.

2. The clinician *reasonably believes* that the person lacks capacity and that the treatment or intervention that they are considering restraining the person to perform is in the person's best interests.

3. The clinician *reasonably believes* the treatment or intervention they are considering restraining the person in order to perform is necessary to prevent harm to that person.

4. The restraint is a *proportionate response* to the likelihood of the person the clinician is restraining suffering harm and how serious that harm is likely to be (sections 5(1) and 6(2)–(3) of the Mental Capacity Act 2005).

Proportionality and what is the least restrictive option are the key considerations that should be in the paramedic's mind. Is the intervention proportionate to the risk to this patient's well-being? Is it the least restrictive option? An example of where restraint is acceptable is a patient with sepsis who is combative, clearly extremely confused, unwell, has no indication of past wishes and feelings that suggest they would not want to receive treatment, and treatment is not futile. Using a blanket wrap and carry chair to restrain the patient and remove them from their property is a proportionate intervention to the risk of them dying from sepsis.

Conversely, consider a patient with dementia who has a laceration that would benefit from sutures. The decision is made that it is in their best interests to be taken to hospital for treatment, but when they are asked to come to hospital, they get very agitated and upset. It is unlikely that using restraint to take the patient to the ED is the least restrictive option; conservative treatment with a bandage may be appropriate, combined with a referral to the district nurses the following day for wound care.

✴ Case Study: Ms F

A 999 call comes in at 16:30 for Ms F, a 75-year-old female whose daughter has come to see her, as she does every Sunday. Normally Ms F is able to answer the door herself and let her daughter in; however, on this occasion, she has not answered the door and her daughter has had to use the key safe to gain entry to the property. She finds Ms F sitting in the living room; she is unkempt and has an odour that suggests she hasn't been managing with her personal care. She is also very confused, thinking it is Friday morning and querying why her daughter has come to visit.

An ambulance is dispatched and on arrival the paramedics are concerned that Ms F has an infection; she is pyrexic, tachycardic and slightly hypotensive, and she is also unable to get out of her chair independently. Her daughter reports that this is very unusual and is very concerned. The paramedics advise Ms F that she may need to attend hospital; she tells them to get lost and lashes out at them.

A capacity assessment is completed and it is clear that Ms F lacks capacity. Her daughter is also surprised that Ms F is refusing treatment as 'she normally does whatever the doctor says, this is very out of character for her'. The paramedics consider that Ms F needs to attend hospital for assessment and possibly intravenous antibiotics. There are no less restrictive options available that are appropriate and Ms F is not likely to regain capacity without treatment. There is also no lasting power of attorney, written statement of wishes or advance decision to refuse treatment.

Following their decision that it is in Ms F's best interests to attend hospital, the paramedics decide that they will need to use a blanket wrap to restrain Ms F and prevent her from lashing out at them. They use the carry chair and two blankets to restrain Ms F and remove her from the property; they then transfer her onto the stretcher. Once in the ambulance, they review the situation and see if Ms F still needs to be restrained. Ms F is still very agitated, so they decide it is appropriate to continue to restrain her until they get to hospital.

When completing their paperwork, the paramedics ensure that they document their capacity assessment, best interests assessment and that they restrained Ms F, including the review of that restraint once she was in the ambulance.

Documenting Ms F's Best Interests Assessment

When documenting Ms F's best interests assessment, it is important that the paramedics demonstrate that they have followed the statutory framework for assessing best interests. They should document:

- that the decision cannot wait because Ms F is not going to regain capacity;
- that there is no advance statement or advance decision to refuse treatment available that refers to the decision;
- who they have consulted to assist them with making the decision (in this example, Ms F's daughter);
- if there is a lasting power of attorney for health or welfare and if they have been consulted (if they have not been contacted, document why this is the case – a reasonable attempt should be made to contact them); and
- that there is no appropriate less restrictive option available.

Documenting Restraint

Any restraint must be documented. This also includes the threat of force and should cover:

- why restraint was required
- what restraint was used
- how long it was used for
- if the restraint was reviewed.

Appropriate Use of the Mental Capacity Act and the Mental Health Act

Paramedics attending patients experiencing a mental health crisis may feel that conveyance to either the ED or a place of safety is required. Just like other patient cohorts, mental health patients may decline treatment or conveyance. Sometimes it will be appropriate to respect the person's wishes and not provide them with any treatment or conveyance to the ED. On other occasions, it may be that providing treatment, conveyance for treatment or conveyance to a place of safety in the absence of patient consent is appropriate; however, this must be done legally and an understanding of the legislative frameworks that relate to mental health patients is essential.

Following amendment in 2007, the Mental Health Act 1983 still allows a more paternalistic approach towards patients with mental disorders than the wider population – for example, mental health patients are one of the only patient groups that can be detained for assessment or treatment without their consent. This is commonly referred to as sectioning. However, the The Mental Capacity Act Code of Practice states:

> The fact that someone has a mental disorder is never sufficient grounds for any compulsory measure to be taken under the Act. Compulsory measures are permitted only where specific criteria about the potential consequences of a person's mental disorder are met. There are many forms of mental disorder which are unlikely to call for compulsory measures. (Department of Health 2015, 2.6)

What the Code is essentially saying here is that it is not appropriate to use the sectioning powers of the Mental Health Act 1983 just because a patient is suffering a mental disorder. As with the Mental Capacity Act 2005, the interventions must be proportionate to the patient's presentation.

In different situations, the Mental Health Act 1983 or the Mental Capacity Act 2005 will be the most appropriate framework to apply to the situation. If a person is suffering from a mental disorder in a public place and needs to be taken to hospital or a place of safety but is refusing, section 136 of the Mental Health Act 1983 will often be the appropriate route to take if the relevant criteria apply, although the Mental Capacity Act 2005 may also be used in certain circumstances (under section 4B, for life-sustaining treatment or a vital act) . If the person in question is in their own property, the Mental Health Act 1983 should be used and a warrant obtained under section 135 to allow a constable to enter the premises for the purpose of removing a mentally disordered person to a place of safety; unless section 4B of the Mental Capacity Act applies.

When assessing the capacity of a patient suffering from a mental disorder, it is likely that it is the ability to use and weigh up information that will be one of the key elements. Some mental disorders are considered to prevent those who have the disorder from having capacity in relation to a specific decision – for example, some patients with anorexia nervosa may be unable to use and weigh up information about the consequences of not eating, despite being able to understand and retain the information (Office of the Public Guardian 2013, 4.22).

If a patient is suffering from a mental disorder, the Mental Capacity Act 2005 can be used to provide treatment for their mental disorder providing they lack capacity, the treatment is in their best interests and the treatment is not regulated by Part 4 of the

Mental Health Act 1983. Part 4 treatments require specific criteria to be met and do not fall under the paramedic scope of practice (Department of Health 2015, 13.31). Treatment under the Mental Health Act 1983 only applies to treatment for the mental disorder from which a patient is suffering and can be given in the absence of their consent (section 63 of the Mental Health Act 1983).

As with any other patient group, treatment can be given for physical illness or injury that is in the best interests of a person suffering from a mental disorder, as long as they lack capacity – for example, treatment for an overdose or self-harm. What the Mental Capacity Act 2005 cannot be used for is as a shortcut to avoid sectioning under the Mental Health Act 1983 for assessment or treatment in hospital for a mental disorder where a patient lacking capacity is refusing, and the section 4B of the Mental Capacity Act 2005 requirement that the treatment, is for life-sustaining treatment, or a vital act, does not apply (*R (Sessay) v SLAM and Commissioner of the Police for the Metropolis* (2011)).

R (Sessay) v SLAM and Commissioner of the Police for the Metropolis (2011)

Background

The police were called regarding concerns about the way in which the claimant (S) had been caring for her child. Upon arrival, the two officers who attended were concerned for S's mental well-being and, considering her to be mentally disordered, took her to hospital under section 5 of the Mental Capacity Act 2005. Upon arrival, S was left in the 136 suite because the staff believed her to be under section 136 of the Mental Health Act 1983; she was detained for 13 hours while an application for admission under section 2 of the Mental Health Act 1983 was made. The Court held that she had been deprived of her liberty/falsely imprisoned, in breach of Article 5 of the European Convention on Human Rights. It was considered that there is a 'complete statutory code covering persons in [S's] . . . position': for the purposes of an emergency situation where the person needed admission for assessment, sections 2, 4 and 135 of the Mental Health Act 1983 should be used.

The Judgement

In our judgement:

i) Part II of the Mental Health Act 1983 provides a comprehensive code for compulsory admission to hospital for non-compliant incapacitated patients such as the Claimant. The common law principle of necessity does not apply in this context.

The Claimant's detention at the hospital on 7 August 2010 was unlawful and in breach of her rights under Article 5 ECHR. The Claimant is entitled to a

---

(continued)

declaration to this effect, together with damages for breach of Article 5 and for false imprisonment to be assessed, if not agreed (para 59).

Application to Paramedic Practice

Based on the facts given, S had no pressing *medical* need secondary to her mental disorder which meant that the use of sections 5 and 6 of the Mental Capacity Act 2005 was appropriate. The police should have got in contact with an Approved Mental Health Professional (AMHP) who would have been able to consider if admission under section was appropriate and organise the appropriate section.

The Mental Health Act 1983 Code of Practice gives guidance on when an application for detention (sectioning) a patient might be appropriate (Department of Health 2015, 14.3–14.13).

Unless you can justify that the deprivation of your patient's liberty is required for the provision of life-sustaining treatment, or a vital act, it is unlikely that taking them to hospital when they are refusing under sections 5–6 of the Mental Capacity Act 2005 would be found to be lawful. In situations where it is believed that a mentally disordered patient is in need of detention (sectioning), it is advisable to contact the social services Emergency Duty Team, or equivalent, and ask to speak to the duty AMHP.

It is essential that paramedics recognise that the detention, or deprivation of liberty, of someone suffering from a mental disorder is always a potential breach of their human rights unless it is done within the appropriate legal framework. Even then, it is essential that the principles of the Mental Capacity Act 2005 and the overarching principles outlined in the Mental Health Act Code of Practice are taken into consideration, and that the least restrictive option is always sought, with detention, or deprivation of liberty, always treated as the last option (section 1 of the Mental Capacity Act 2005; Department of Health 2015, 1.1).

The Future

There have been criticisms of both the Mental Capacity Act 2005 and the Mental Health Act 1983. The Mental Capacity Act 2005 is considered not to have sufficient safeguards built in for the use of restraint or force. The safeguards that have been put in place for when restraint is considered to amount to a deprivation of liberty are considered to be inadequate and in need of review (this was completed by the Law Commission in 2017, which suggested that the Deprivation of Liberty safeguards are replaced by the Liberty Protection Safeguards) (Law Commission 2017; Szmukler 2018, p. 86).

The Mental Health Act 1983 is considered by some to discriminate against those with mental disorders and to be at odds with the United Nations Convention on the Right of Persons with Disabilities (Hale 2017). This is because the legislation does not allow those with a mental disorder to enjoy the same rights as those with a physical disorder.

The justification for this disparity between the respect for autonomy and rights of those with mental and physical health disorders is the risk of harm. Broadly, if a person has a mental disorder and is a risk to themselves or others, this could be sufficient justification for detention and involuntary treatment (Szmukler 2018). This is supported by Article 5(1)(e) of the European Convention on Human Rights:

> No one shall be deprived of his liberty save in the following cases and in accordance with a procedure prescribed by law: (e) the lawful detention . . . of persons of unsound mind, alcoholics or drug addicts or vagrants.

In practice, this means that those with a mental disorder may be given treatment even when they retain the capacity to refuse.

There is sometimes a nervousness to use force to treat a patient in the absence of a clear statutory authority, such as the Mental Health Act 1983 (i.e. formally sectioning a patient for assessment or treatment). This nervousness may mean that a patient refusing treatment who lacks capacity does not receive treatment that is in their best interests because it is easier to treat them with a presumption of capacity and capacitous refusal of treatment (Szmukler 2018, p. 87). It also means that in some circumstances, the Mental Health Act 1983 may be used inappropriately for those who lack capacity, do not have a mental disorder of a 'traditional nature', but require force in order to be given treatment (Szmukler 2018, pp. 86–87).

The 'Fusion' Approach

Szmukler (2018, p. 83) offers a case for a new law that would not discriminate against those with mental disorder. He suggests a move towards a new 'fusion' approach, a generic law that combines the Mental Health Act 1983 and the Mental Capacity Act 2005. This would create a capacity-based law that combines the emphasis of autonomy that is central to the Mental Capacity Act 2005 with the clearly regulated use of detention and force found in the Mental Health Act 1983.

The proposed law has similar core principles to the Mental Capacity Act 2005 and borrows heavily from its diagnostic and functional tests; the definition of 'best interests' is also similar to the Mental Capacity Act 2005, but with a stronger emphasis on the participation of the person in making the decision (Szmukler, 2018, p. 89).

Where a person is objecting to treatment, the fusion law demands that a set of conditions are met. If any of the conditions are no longer met, the person must be discharged:

1. *The person has an impairment or dysfunction of the mind.*

2. *The person lacks capacity to make a decision about his or her care or treatment.*

3. *The person needs care or treatment in his or her best interests.*

4. *The person objects to the proposed care or treatment.*

5. *The proposed objective cannot be achieved in a less restrictive fashion.* (Szmuckler 2018, p. 90).

In an emergency, paramedics (and other professionals), with a reasonable belief that a person lacks capacity would be able to intervene and take the person to an appropriate place for assessment (Szmuckler 2018, p. 90). The following would then be instigated:

1. An emergency assessment, including capacity assessment, and an immediately required treatment period would follow, lasting only 24 hours (second opinion and consultation with those involved in best interests decision making would be required for an extension of this) (Szmuckler 2018, p. 91).

2. If it was decided that further involuntary treatment was required, a care plan would be made and shared with the patient, and treatment would continue for up to 28 days (Szmuckler 2018, p. 91).

3. If the involuntary treatment was required for more than 28 days, this would be authorised by a tribunal (Szmuckler 2018, p. 91).

Involuntary treatment could also be provided to those lacking capacity for the protection of others; this would be subject to it being in the patient's best interests (for example, where they are being aggressive towards someone they love and to whom are not normally aggressive) or where treatment in the patient's best interests caused a risk to others (for example, being aggressive towards other in-patients) (Szmuckler 2018, p. 91).

Szmuckler's 'fusion law' proposal would also apply to offenders (those in the criminal justice system) with an impairment in their mental functioning; however, this will not be discussed here.

If implemented, the fusion law proposal would provide paramedics and other healthcare professionals with a clear statutory framework to work within and would remove some of the challenges faced by the emergency services when working with the cognitively impaired, such as the previously discussed 'Sessay problem' (*R (Sessay) v SLAM and Commissioner of the Police for the Metropolis (2011)*).

Summary

The Mental Capacity Act 2005 provides a statutory framework for the assessment of capacity and for making decisions for those who lack capacity. Central to the Act is the promotion of autonomy, with case law continuing to emphasise this by increasing the weight being given to the person's past wishes and feelings when they lack capacity. The Mental Capacity Act 2005 is not perfect and fails to provide adequate safeguards that are found in other legislation that authorises involuntary treatment, such as the Mental Health Act 1983. A 'fusion law' would reduce discrimination against those with mental disorders and would provide safeguards to ensure that involuntary treatment is not given arbitrarily.

> **Tips for Practice**
>
> - Capacity is time- and decision-specific; you should always ensure that the decision cannot wait until the person regains capacity and that the treatment option that you choose is the least restrictive one.
> - Clear documentation of your capacity assessment, best interests decision-making process and any restraint used is essential.
> - The Mental Health Act 1983 should be used instead of the Mental Capacity Act 2005 where the person being assessed is not suffering from any physical illness, but only psychiatric illness.

Recommended Reading

Szmukler, G (2018) *Men in White Coats: Treatment under Coercion*. Oxford: Oxford University Press.

References

39 Essex Chambers (2014) *Heart of England NHS Trust v JB*. Available at: www.39essex.com/cop_cases/heart-of-england-nhs-foundation-trust-v-jb.

39 Essex Chambers (2015) *Wye Valley NHS Trust v Mr B*. Available at: www.39essex.com/cop_cases/wye-valley-nhs-trust-v-mr-b.

39 Essex Chambers (2016) *A brief guide to carrying out capacity assessments*. Available at: www.39essex.com/content/wp-content/uploads/2016/08/Capacity-Assessments-Guide-August-2016.pdf.

Braye, S and Preston-Shoot, M (2017) *Learning from SARs: A Report for the London Safeguarding Adults Board*. Available at: http://londonadass.org.uk/wp-content/uploads/2014/12/London-SARs-Report-Final-Version.pdf.

Cooper, A and White, E (eds) (2017) *Safeguarding Adults under the Care Act 2014: Understanding Good Practice*. London: Jessica Kingsley.

Department of Health (2015) *Mental Health Act 1983: Code of Practice*. London: The Stationery Office.

Hale, B (2017) *Mental Health Law*. London: Sweet & Maxwell.

Harris, J (1985) *The Value of Life: An Introduction to Medical Ethics*. London: Routledge.

Heywood, R (2014) Revisiting advanced decision making under the Mental Capacity Act 2005: a tale of mixed messages. *Medical Law Review*, 23(1): 88–102.

House of Lords (2015) *Mental Capacity Act 2005: Post-legislative Scrutiny*. London: The Stationery Office.

Jackson, E (2016) *Medical Law: Text, Cases, and Materials*. Oxford: Oxford University Press.

Law Commission (2017) *Mental Capacity and Deprivation of Liberty*. London: Williams Lea Group.

National Institute for Health and Care Excellence (NICE) (2017) *Stroke and transient ischaemic attack in over 16s: diagnosis and initial management*. Available at: www.nice.org.uk/guidance/cg68/chapter/1-guidance.

Office of the Public Guardian (2013) *Mental Capacity Act Code of Practice*. London: The Stationery Office.

Szmukler, G (2018) *Men in White Coats: Treatment under Coercion*. Oxford: Oxford University Press.

UK Cases

Aintree University Hospitals NHS Foundation Trust v James [2014] 1 AC 591

Heart of England NHS Trust v JB [2014] EWHC 342 (COP)

R (Sessay) v SLAM and Commissioner of the Police for the Metropolis [2011] EWHC 2617

Re C (Adult: Refusal of Treatment) [1994] 1 WLR 290

Re MB (Adult: Medical Treatment) [1997] 38 BMLR 175

Re T (Adult: Refusal of Treatment) [1993] Fam 95

Wye Valley NHS Trust v Mr B [2015] EWCOP 60

EU Cases

Herczegfalvy v Austria (1993) 15 EHRR 437

UK Legislation

Adults with Incapacity (Scotland) Act 2000

Human Rights Act 1998

Mental Capacity Act 2005

Mental Capacity Act (Northern Ireland) 2016

Mental Health Act 1983

Mental Health (Care and Treatment) (Scotland) Act 2003

Chapter 11

Legal and Ethical Principles in the Treatment of Children

Will Broughton and Georgette Eaton

Introduction

Healthcare professionals caring for children and young people have a number of ethical and legal obligations with which they should be familiar, and these are often outlined in best practice guidance, statute and case law. The Health and Care Professions Council (HCPC) offers no specific advice in relation to children and, other than inclusion on the undergraduate curriculum, nor does the College of Paramedics (College of Paramedics 2017). With those aged 0–14 estimated to make up just 18.4% of the UK population (Statistics Portal 2018), it seems that an ageing population has almost moved children off the agenda.

The place of children in medical law is frequently the subject of much contention, often associated with ethical dilemmas. This is far from an easy subject for any healthcare professional, regardless of their education or experience. When professionals encounter these difficult situations, they should be reassured by the publications that are in place to support them, but must also seek guidance from those who know the publications in detail.

When making decisions about the healthcare of children and young people, there are a number of essential principles outlined by the British Medical Association (2016, p. 5): *All children and young people can expect the following:*

- *To be kept as fully informed as they wish, and as is possible, about their care and treatment.*

- *Health professionals to act as advocates.*

- *To have their views and wishes sought and taken into account as part of promoting their welfare in the widest possible sense.*

- *To be the individual who consents to assessment or treatment when they are competent to do so.*

- *To be encouraged to take decisions in collaboration with other family members, especially parents, if this is feasible.*

- *To be able to expect that information provided will remain confidential unless there are exceptional reasons that require confidentiality to be breached.*

This chapter will set out some key pieces of guidance, legislation, case law and statutes with which professionals should be familiar in order to practise safely. It includes profession-specific guidance for clinical practice. These should be read in conjunction with the Recommended Reading that has been identified at the end of the chapter, which serves as a point of reference for those interested in the law and ethics relating to paediatric paramedic practice.

The Rights and Interests of Children

Within the UK, there are several main Acts that govern the legal rights of children and exist to protect their interests.

England and Wales

The Children Act 1989 allocates duties to parents, local authorities, courts and other agencies in the UK to ensure that the welfare of children is promoted and that they are safeguarded as appropriate. The Act outlines that the child's welfare is of paramount importance and that the views of the child must be respected.

This Act centres on the idea that children are best cared for within their own families, but it also makes provision for those who cannot co-operate with statutory bodies. It outlines exactly who would have parental responsibility or guardianship of the child and allows anyone with parental responsibility to act alone – so decisions may be based on one parent.

Although mostly aimed at court decisions for care, the Act produces a list of general principles that are pertinent to clinical practice in order to maximally promote and protect the child's general welfare and ensure that any action taken is in their best interests. These principles are as follows and should be considered:

- The wishes and feelings of the child.
- The physical, emotional and educational needs of the child.
- The likely effect on the child of any change in circumstances.
- Any harm which the child is at risk of suffering or has suffered.
- How capable the child's parents or guardians are in terms of meeting the child's needs.
- The relevant characteristics of the child, including their age, gender and background.

The Children Act 2004 supplemented the 1989 Act and reinforced the message that all organisations working with children have a duty to help safeguard and promote the welfare of children.

The Family Law Reform Act 1969 is largely concerned with the law relating to the age of majority (where a person shall attain full age on becoming 18 years old), the property rights of illegitimate children, the provision of blood tests to confirm paternity and other provisions in connection with registration of the birth of an illegitimate child. The Act also makes it quite clear that those who are aged 16–17 have the same legal ability to consent to any medical, surgical or dental treatment as anyone above the age of 18, without the consent from their parent or guardian.

Northern Ireland

The Children (Northern Ireland) Order 1995

This is the principal statute governing the care, upbringing and protection of children in Northern Ireland. It affects all those who work and care for children, whether they are parents, paid carers or volunteers. This Order brought together most of the 'public' and 'private' law relating to children in a single statutory framework along the lines of the Children Act 1989 in England and Wales. The legislative framework for Northern Ireland's child protection system is set out in this, the Children (Northern Ireland) Order 1995.

The Children's Services Co-operation Act (Northern Ireland) 2015 builds on this and requires public authorities (including health services) to co-operate in contributing to the well-being of children and young people in the areas of:

- physical and mental health
- enjoyment of play and leisure
- learning and achievement
- living conditions, rights and economic well-being.

The Age of Majority Act (Northern Ireland) 1969

Under section 4 of the Age of Majority Act (Northern Ireland) 1969, patients aged 16 or 17 can provide consent to their own medical care if they are deemed to be capable of making informed decisions

Scotland

The Children (Scotland) Act 1995

Under this Act, mothers and married fathers have automatic parental responsibilities and rights (section 3). Unmarried fathers can acquire parental responsibilities and rights by entering into an agreement with the mother or by application to the court. Regarding children born on or after 4 May 2006, fathers who register the birth jointly with the mother will also acquire parental responsibilities and rights.

The Law Reform (Parent and Child) (Scotland) Act 1986

When parents separate or divorce, or indeed have always lived apart, much of the legal framework relevant to their parenting issues can be found in this Act. Importantly, this Act expresses that the child has a right to have any views they wish to express taken into account, in light of the child's age and maturity, in relation to whom the child lives with.

The Age of Legal Capacity (Scotland) Act 1991 (the 'Scottish Act')

Under the 'Scottish Act', the age of majority (adulthood) is considered to be the sixteenth birthday. Also outlined in the Act are certain circumstances in which a person under the age of 16 is deemed to have the capacity to consent to any dental, medical or surgical procedure, with the proviso that they are capable of understanding the nature and consequences of the proposed intervention.

Parental Responsibility

In England, Wales and Northern Ireland, parental responsibilities may be exercised until a young person reaches the age of 18.

In Scotland, only the aspect of parental responsibilities concerned with the giving of 'guidance' endures until the age of 18 – guidance meaning the provision of advice. The rest is lost when a young person reaches the age of 16, although some may be lost before this if the child attains legal capacity to act on their own behalf.

Throughout the UK, a mother will automatically gain parental responsibility at birth. The parental responsibility held by others will vary according to the place of birth and when the birth is registered. In *England and Wales*, a father will have parental responsibility if he is married to the child's mother when the child is born or if they have jointly adopted the child. If married parents later divorce, they both still retain parental responsibility. For unmarried parents, they must either jointly register the birth (from 1 December 2003), put in place a parental responsibility agreement with the mother or obtain a parental responsibility order from a court. In *Scotland*, a father has parental responsibility if he is married to the mother when the child is conceived or they become married at any point after conception. An unmarried father must be named on the birth certificate to gain parental responsibility (from 4 May 2006). In *Northern Ireland*, a father has parental responsibility if he is married to the mother at the time of the child's birth. If a father marries the mother after the birth, he will still have parental responsibility if he lives in Northern Ireland at the time of the marriage. An unmarried father has parental responsibility if he is named, or becomes named, on the child's birth certificate (from 15 April 2002).

Same-sex partners will both have parental responsibility if they were civil partners or were married at the time of donor insemination or fertility treatment. For same-sex partners who are not civil partners or married, the second parent may obtain parental responsibility by applying to the court if a parental agreement was made or by becoming a civil partner/husband/wife of the other parent and making a parental responsibility agreement or jointly registering the birth.

Consent

A child or young person is classed as under the age of 16 in Scotland and 18 in England, Wales and Northern Ireland. As outlined above, capacity to consent to medical treatment for children aged 16–17 is presumed within each nation of the UK, unless the patient does not pass the assessment outlined by the Mental Capacity Act 2005. The *Mental Health Act 1983: Code of Practice* (2015) offers guidance for those with parental responsibility, as well as on assessing the competence of children and the capacity of children and young people when making decisions about their admission and/or treatment.

In order to give consent to the medical treatment of a child or young person, that person must be:

- a competent child or young person, giving consent for their own care;
- a parent or other person or agency with parental responsibility where the decision is in the best interests of the child;
- a court;
- an appointed proxy (in Scotland where the patient is over the age of 16 and is unable to make decisions for themselves); or
- a person caring for a child – for example, a grandparent or child minder – and who may do what is reasonable in the circumstances to safeguard or promote the child's welfare (British Medical Association 2016; Royal College of Nursing 2017).

Despite extensive legal guidance, there is no discussion concerning the capacity of children under the age of 16 or capacity for the refusal of treatment. Such decisions are governed by common law, as demonstrated below.

Gillick Competence and Fraser Guidelines

Perhaps the most notorious aspect of law within the UK associated with children is that of *Gillick* and Fraser. It is important to note that these are related, but not interchangeable, terms.

Gillick competence refers to the assessment that could be made in relation to whether a child under the age of 16 has the capacity to consent to treatment without parental or guardian consent. This is relevant in England, Wales and Northern Ireland.

This was a landmark decision which raised a number of complex legal issues. The House of Lords was called upon to resolve the extent of the parental right to control a minor child and when – and indeed whether – such a minor could receive contraceptive advice, or consent to medical treatment, against the wishes or knowledge of their parents. Finally, it fell to be determined whether a doctor, in exercising their clinical duty, would be guilty of a criminal offence by providing contraception or advice to underage patients.

As *Gillick* was decided in the House of Lords, its authority extends to the whole of the UK. However, subsequent Scottish law has superseded *Gillick* with the enactment of the 'Scottish Act'.

Gillick v West Norfolk & Wisbech Area Health Authority (1986)

The Facts of the Case

Mrs Gillick was a mother of (at that time) four children and raised concerns about guidance issued by the Department of Health and Social Security surrounding the provision of contraceptive advice and treatment for a girl under the age of 16, when at that age the girl could not lawfully consent to intercourse. Mrs Gillick sought a declaration from the court that the Department's guidance was unlawful as it adversely interfered with parental rights and duties.

The Judgement

The application for a declaration was dismissed. Parental rights, as such, did not exist, except insofar as necessary to safeguard the best interests of a minor. In some circumstances, a minor would be able to give consent in their own right without the knowledge or approval of their parents. The test proposed by Lord Scarman posits that a minor will be able to consent to treatment if they demonstrate 'sufficient understanding and intelligence to understand fully what is proposed' ([1986] AC 112, 187[D]). The test is now often referred to as '*Gillick* competence' and is an integral aspect of medical law.

Fraser guidelines refer to Lord Fraser's involvement with the *Gillick* case. Lord Fraser commented on the responsibility of doctors to ensure adequate capacity of children specifically receiving contraceptive advice and prescriptions. He stated that a doctor could proceed to give advice and treatment:
Provided they are satisfied with the following criteria:

1. *That the girl (although under the age of 16) will understand his advice;*

2. *That he cannot persuade her to inform her parents or to allow him to inform the parents that she is seeking contraceptive advice;*

3. *That she is very likely to continue having sexual intercourse with or without contraceptive treatment;*

4. *That unless she receives contraceptive advice or treatment her physical or mental health are both likely to suffer;*

5. *That her best interests require him to give her contraceptive advice, treatment or both without the parental consent.*

These guidelines are accepted by the Department of Health in England, Wales and Northern Ireland. There is no specific government guidance from Scotland.

> **Pause for Thought**
>
> *It is important to note that Fraser does not comment on the capacity of children for any other treatment or procedure.*

Since these rulings, *Gillick* and Fraser have become interchangeable terms across medical communities as a means to assessing competence in children. This is, as we can see, incorrect. Wheeler (2006, p. 332) argues that if *Gillick* became completely incorporated into Fraser, the detailed assessment of the child's capacity provided by the original case would be lost. Likewise, if Fraser became completely synonymous with *Gillick*, Lord Fraser's comments on the particular clinical problem of contraceptives in girls under the age of 16 would be lost in the generalities of children's capacity.

Although the focus in *Gillick* was on the provision of contraceptives, the principles of this have applied to the consent of minors to other forms of treatment. *Gillick* was unsuccessfully challenged in *R (Axon) v Secretary of State for Health* (2006), where guidance for abortion under the age of 16 from the Department of Health was challenged by parents.

Children under the Age of 16 Who are Not *Gillick* Competent

The Children Act 1989 outlines that consent for treatment of non-*Gillick* competent children is by parents or those with parental responsibility. Parental responsibility is defined in the Act as comprising the authority, duties, rights, responsibilities and powers which parents have in relation to their children (section 3(1)). This also includes consent to medical treatment on behalf of the child. Parental responsibility may be acquired by relatives, guardians, local authorities or the court.

Normally, the consent of one person with parental responsibility will suffice for the purposes of medical treatment. This is outlined in *Re R (A Minor) (Wardship: Consent to Treatment)* (1992), where the Court of Appeal demonstrated that a *Gillick* competent adolescent had the ability to consent to treatment, though should the adolescent refuse the treatment, consent could be given by someone else who had parental responsibility over the child, such as the Court. Essentially, refusal by a *Gillick* competent child may be overridden if consent for treatment is obtained from a valid source.

16–17-Year-Olds Who Lack Mental Capacity

There may also be occasions when a 16–17-year-old, who would usually be presumed to be competent to make decisions, may lack mental capacity or may become incapacitated. In such circumstances, healthcare professionals need to review the detailed guidance within the Mental Capacity Act 2005 (see Chapter 10 in this book) and seek expert advice.

In England and Wales, the Mental Capacity Act 2005 outlines the principle that any decision or action taken must be in the best interests of the 16–17-year-old who lacks capacity. However, there are some provisions in the Act that do not apply to 16–17-year-olds:

- They cannot make a Lasting Power of Attorney (LPA).
- They cannot make an Advance Decision to Refuse Treatment.
- The Court of Protection cannot make a statutory will.

In Scotland, the Adults with Incapacity (Scotland) Act 2000 sets out the framework for regulating intervention in the affairs of adults (people over the age of 16) who have impaired capacity. It allows people over the age of 16 who have capacity to appoint a welfare attorney to make health and personal welfare decisions once their capacity is lost. The Court of Session may also appoint a deputy to make these decisions.

In Northern Ireland, treatment can be provided in the young person's best interests if a parent cannot be contacted, although healthcare professionals should seek additional legal advice if applying for non-emergency interventions (General Medical Council 2007). There are also plans to introduce new legislation relating to both mental health and mental capacity in Northern Ireland; however, currently there are no publications concerning this.

Refusal of Treatment

Just because a child or young person is able to consent and demonstrate competence may not allow the right to refuse treatment to be exercised. In England, Wales and Northern Ireland, a competent refusal can be overruled by a court or a person with parental responsibility. In *Re W (A Minor) (Medical Treatment: Court Justification)* (1993), the English Court of Appeal ordered that a 16-year-old girl under the care of the local authority suffering with anorexia nervosa be transferred against her will to a hospital specialising in eating disorders. Her argument was the presumption of capacity under the Family Law Reform Act 1969 that allowed her to refuse treatment in the same way as an adult. The claim was unsuccessful and the Court further held that the Family Law Reform Act 1969 is inapplicable to the issue of whether a 16-year-old minor has the absolute right to refuse medical treatment. Essentially, even if a child is *Gillick* competent or has reached the age of 16, the right to refuse treatment for life-threatening conditions has been rejected by the Court, usually on the grounds that capacity needs to be considered very carefully and in the context of a particular circumstance or decision. Generally, the graver the decision, the greater the capacity required in order to make that decision. This is illustrated by three cases where life-saving blood transfusions were refused by children who were Jehovah's Witnesses (*Re S (A Minor) (Consent to Medical Treatment)* (1994); *Re A (A Minor) (Wardship: Medical Treatment)* (1993); and *Re L (Medical Treatment: Gillick Competency)* (1998)).

✳ Case Study

You are a critical care paramedic working for an English Helicopter Emergency Medical Service (HEMS). You are dispatched to a multiple vehicle road traffic collision on a busy motorway. Various resources are already on scene and you are requested to attend a 14-year-old boy who has been ejected from the car he was travelling in and has sustained a partial amputation above the knee. Two other people in the car are fatalities. On your arrival, two tourniquets have already been applied to the leg, which continues to bleed. The boy is conscious but haemodynamically compromised and in pain. On handover from the paramedic on scene, you are told that he is refusing blood or plasma products due to his religion, and only consents to pain relief.

What do you do?

The issue with refusal of treatment is not the lack of rights for a child or young person to refuse, but rather that the refusal of consent by one holder of the rights (the child) is ineffectual against the willingness of another (a court or a parent) to consent, especially if this results in the competent minor having a more limited right of self-determination than the competent adult. Such a view is considered to be incompatible with Article 8 of the Human Rights Act 1998.

Consent in an Emergency

In an emergency, where consent is unavailable – for example, when the patient is unable to communicate their wishes and where nobody with parental responsibility is available – it is legally and ethically appropriate for health professionals to proceed with treatment necessary to preserve the life, health or well-being of the patient. In extreme situations, health professionals are advised to take all essential steps to stabilise the patient. Legal advice may be needed once emergency action has been taken, and care should be taken to document every conversation and action that took place following a decision to proceed without consent.

> **Pause for Thought.**
>
> *An emergency is best described as a situation where the requirement for treatment is so pressing that there is not time to refer the matter to the court.*

Parental and Medical Disagreement

On occasion, parents and medical professionals will disagree regarding the treatment of children. This may be down to conflicting cultural or religious expectations, different values concerning the concept of life or simply to a lack of understanding on both sides. Whilst such differences of opinion are not uncommon, usually a solution can easily be found.

Generally, as was demonstrated in *Re B (A Minor) (Wardship: Medical Treatment)* (1990), the courts are willing to override parental refusal if the treatment is considered to be in the best interests of the child. As with *Re A (Children) (Conjoined Twins: Surgical Separation)* (2001), even if the views of the parents are considered sincere and reasonable, the court outlined the principle that parental views are not necessarily determinative. However, in *Glass v UK* (2004), the European Court of Human Rights (ECtHR) confirmed that disputes about best interests decisions between those with parental responsibility and medical staff required referral to the court for adjudication. In this case, where the doctor's actions had bypassed parental consent, there was held to be a violation of Article 8 (the right to family life) and the hospital had a duty to involve the patient in decisions relating to their treatment.

The court also tends to favour decisions that preserve life, although in *Re T (A Minor) (Wardship: Medical Treatment)* (1997), it was held that a loving parent's decision not to treat a child who suffered from a life-threatening disease was not to be interfered with, as they had made an assessment of what was in their child's best interests.

Disagreements regarding the continued treatment of children also occur. In *Re Wyatt (A Child) (Medical Treatment: Continuation of Order)* (2005), considerable weight was given to the medical evidence to withdraw treatment from the child, Charlotte Wyatt, against the wishes of her parents.

The recent case of *Yates and Gard v Great Ormond Street Hospital for Children NHS Foundation Trust* (2017) was a powerful example of a parent's wish to offer their child every opportunity for medical treatment, despite the advice of medical professionals. The case was complex and went through multiple legal challenges, including the ECtHR, before the Honourable Justice Francis gave a final ruling in July 2017 that 'Charlie's life cannot be improved and that the only remaining course is for him to be given palliative care and to permit him to die with dignity'. Ultimately, the decision was made in the best interests of the child, but demonstrates the possibility as well as the ramifications of legal challenge when there is disagreement between parents and medical professionals. The UK saw another complex case in 2018, *James and Evans v Alder Hey Children's NHS Foundation Trust* (2018). This case endured a lengthy legal challenge and attracted a great deal of media attention. In *Yates and Gard v Great Ormond Street Hospital for Children NHS Foundation Trust* (2017), McFarlane LJ observed: 'As the authorities to which I have already made reference underline again and again, the sole principle is that the best interests of the child must prevail and that must apply even to cases where parents, for the best of motives, hold on to some alternative view.' What both cases demonstrate is that medical professionals and parents are entitled to challenge the views of one another in relation to the care of a child. When, despite the process of mediation, no consensus is able to be reached, the matter should then be referred to the courts for a final decision.

Confidentiality

In medical law and ethics, children can often be a challenging group as much of the legislation does not necessarily relate directly to them, and the legal definition of a child is different between Scotland and the rest of the UK.

As with other principles of confidentiality (see Chapter 5), information about children should also be confidential. One issue that arises in respect of children and confidentiality is whether parents have a right to be informed about medical details relating to their child, and that children may withhold sensitive information from their parents or carers. In *R (Axon) v Secretary of State for Health* (2006), Mrs Axon unsuccessfully challenged guidance for abortion for those under the age of 16 from the Department of Health. She also highlighted that parents should be informed when advice concerning sexual matters was given to children.

The common law is clearer in this by stating that the mature minor's right to confidentiality is permitted when it is deemed in their best interests (*Gillick v West Norfolk & Wisbech Area Health Authority* (1986)). The court held that *Gillick* competent children have the same rights to confidentiality as adults. Following this case, it appears that if a child is not *Gillick* competent, then parents should be informed unless there is a robust reason for not doing so. This may well then come down to the ethical standpoint of the clinician in the situation in which this occurs.

Despite this, there continues to be a duty placed upon the clinician to attempt to persuade the child to inform those who hold parental responsibility, or even to allow them to make contact with the parents themselves.

A breach of confidentiality may also be justified in order to protect children from abuse, as outlined in *A County Council v SB* (2010).

Mental Ill Health in Children

Figures show that in 2015, 2.6% of the English population aged 5–17 received treatment from Child and Adolescent Mental Health Services (CAMHS) (Children's Commissioner for England 2017). A particular problem in cases concerning children with mental ill health is the interplay between mental capacity and mental health legislation.

The use of sections in the Mental Health Act 1983 is not age-restricted. Therefore, if a child is detained under the Act, there is a duty to ensure that the environment is suitable for their age and needs. It is important that a CAMHS assessment is carried out at the earliest opportunity, and the child should be in an environment that facilitates this – this must never be a police station. There is similar guidance in the Mental Health (Wales) Measure 2010.

Section 2 of the Mental Health (Scotland) Act 2015 makes specific provisions to safeguard the welfare of any child under the age of 18. Section 2 requires that any functions under the Act in relation to a child with a mental disorder should be carried out in the way that best secures the welfare of the child. In particular, it is necessary to take into account:

- the wishes and feelings of the child alongside the views of any carers;
- the carers' needs and any circumstances which are considered relevant to the discharge of the child;
- where the child is or has been subject to detention or a compulsory treatment order, the importance of providing appropriate services to that child; and
- the importance of the function being discharged in the manner that appears to involve the minimum restriction on the freedom of the child as is necessary in the circumstances.

In Northern Ireland, children are not within the scope of the Mental Capacity (NI) Act 2016, the newest mental health legislation, and therefore the Mental Health (Northern Ireland) Order 1986 remains the main legislation for children. Purely on the basis of age, those under the age of 16 will not be able to access the range of protections and safeguards outlined in the Mental Capacity (NI) Act 2016 that are afforded to those over the age of 16 who lack capacity as a result of mental illness or disability. Calls to review the impact of the mental health legislation on children in Northern Ireland have been proposed (Northern Ireland Commissioner for Children and Young People 2017). The Children (Northern Ireland) Order 1995 also contains provisions for a court to direct a parent or guardian to bring a child or young person to hospital for assessment of their mental disorder and, if necessary, for treatment (Guidelines and Audit Implementation Network 2011).

Organ Donation

Chapter 13 gives an introductory note on the use of uncontrolled donation after circulatory death, and therefore it seems pertinent to give a brief note regarding organ donation in relation to children here. This concept presents many ethical decisions and conflicts of interest, but an overview of the law in relation to organ donation may assist with this understanding,

Section 2 of the Human Tissue Act 2004 provides that *Gillick* competent children (under the age of 18) can give *appropriate* consent to donate organs. If the child lacks capacity or does not wish to make a decision, section 2(3) outlines how consent can be given by a person with parental responsibility. However, it is the notion of *appropriate* consent that is considered important, as this is considered insufficient without court approval. The court's paramount consideration is the welfare of the donor over that of the recipient (para A11) and children can be considered as living donors in very rare circumstances. In *Hart v Brown* (1972), the court found that the donor's psychological benefit (namely her sister's survival and companionship) was sufficient to allow sibling-to-sibling organ donation.

Fetal Rights

There is considerable legal contention and ethical debate concerning abortion and prenatal life, which is largely beyond the scope of this book. However, it is worth clarifying Fetal rights. A fetus has no legal personality or legal status until it is born and exists independent of its mother (*Paton v British Pregnancy Advisory Service* (1978)). Even if the fetus did have a right to life under Article 2 of the European Convention on Human Rights (which the court refused to assert in *Paton v UK* (1980)), this right would be constrained in the event of the life of the pregnant mother being in jeopardy. This also means that pregnant women with capacity have a right to refuse medical treatment, and this is not outweighed by any rights of the fetus even if it is viable (*St George's Healthcare Trust v S* (1998)). This was also confirmed in *Attorney General's Reference (No 3 of 1994)* (1997), which found that the fetus has no independent legal personality until birth. This is further outlined in *Vo v France* (2005), where the ECtHR found no consensus on the moral status of the fetus, and so the extent of the right to life of the fetus under Article 2 remains undefined.

Use of a Chaperone

When a paramedic is required to treat a child or young person, in most cases a parent or carer will be present and can act as a chaperone for them. However, given the diverse roles in which paramedics may work, many of which include emergency and unscheduled care, it is possible that you will be called to examine a child who may be alone or with other children. A competent child or young person may also state that they do not wish for a parent or carer to be present.

Employing organisations should have a chaperone policy and this should be made available to staff and patients. A patient may request a chaperone and as a medical professional you should be in a position to offer a chaperone when appropriate. However, if offered, a patient also has a right to decline the presence of a chaperone.

The HCPC does not provide any guidance relating to use of chaperones. The General Medical Council (GMC) (2013) states that a chaperone should *usually* be a health professional and that the registrant must be satisfied that the chaperone will:

a) be sensitive and respect the patient's dignity and confidentiality

b) reassure the patient if they show any signs of distress or discomfort

c) be familiar with the procedures involved in a routine intimate examination

d) stay for the whole examination and be able to see what the [doctor] is doing, if practical

e) be prepared to raise concerns if they are concerned about the [doctor's] behaviour or actions.

When considering paramedic practice, a number of issues arise. Paramedics may find themselves in lone working situations and may be required to examine a child. Whilst it is appropriate to use parents or carers, they are unlikely to meet points c), d) and e) in the GMC guidance listed above and be in a position to act as an impartial observer. Therefore, the registrant must consider if the examination is immediately required in order to make decisions about the care of a child or young person. Consideration should also be given to requesting the presence of an appropriately trained adult, alongside the parent or carer. If using a parent or carer, the examination or procedure should be explained so that they understand in advance what it is you will be doing.

If a child or young person declines the presence of a chaperone, consider whether it would be appropriate and necessary to continue. The fact that the patient has been examined without the presence of a chaperone should be recorded alongside a rationale for proceeding with the examination.

The use of chaperones is to protect both the patient and the registered clinician. Paramedics should, wherever possible, ensure that an appropriately trained chaperone is present when examining a child or young person, particularly if that examination is of intimate areas.

✴ Case Study

You are a paramedic working in a rural minor illness and injury unit. You are the only clinician in the building today and there is a receptionist who is booking in patients. A 12-year-old boy presents with two friends complaining of severe pain in his left testicle which came on after being hit in the groin by one of his friends. The patient is booked in by the (female) receptionist and you bring the child into your treatment room accompanied by the friend who hit him (also a 12-year-old boy).

(continued)

The child is in severe discomfort and after confirming some basic details (including allergies) you offer some analgesia, which is accepted by the child. The history is suggestive of testicular torsion as there is recent trauma, followed by unilateral testicular pain that is severe and radiating into the abdomen. The receptionist has been trying to contact the child's parents with the numbers provided, but as yet there has been no answer.

You have requested an ambulance (20 minutes' away) and have successfully referred to the paediatric surgeon at the local hospital, who agrees with your working diagnosis of torsion. As this case involves trauma, you would like to examine the area to rule out any injury that may require immediate attention.

How will you examine this child?

- Chaperone required – the other 12-year-old is not suitable, would not be an impartial observer and may not be a reliable witness.

- The receptionist may be a suitable chaperone, but there are many things to consider: do they have the required training, are they willing to act in this capacity, are they available and would the child be comfortable with a chaperone of a different gender?

- Is the examination going to affect the management of this patient? There is potential, given the nature of the injury, for it to be appropriate to carry out an inspection and examination of the area concerned. You could wait until the ambulance arrives as there will likely be another health professional who could then act as the chaperone.

- A final option to consider is that whilst the examination is indicated, the child could be given space to inspect the site themselves and let you know if there is any injury. If a suitable chaperone is not available and you do not believe the examination to be immediately required, then you could justify waiting until the child is in the care of the hospital team.

Clinical Holding and Using Restraint to Provide Treatment

Clinical holding is not defined by any profession-specific guidance, but it is a recognised method of supporting a child with a painful procedure (Royal College of Nursing 2010). Clinical or therapeutic holding is presented as a method that differs from restraint due to the degree of force required and the intention. What is not defined in the literature is what would constitute a painful procedure, and this creates some difficulty in terms of being able to determine if 'holding' would be appropriate.

Consider the one-year old child who is unwell with a fever and, despite your best intentions, they will not let you take their temperature. Is it appropriate to work with a parent, carer or colleague to 'hold' the child whilst an accurate temperature is recorded? This is a difficult situation in which to provide absolute clarity; however, looking from a purely clinical perspective, the temperature reading may influence your overall management of the child and therefore would be considered an essential observation. The child is not in a position to be able to give consent for holding, nor are they in a position to refuse any examination or intervention. A person with parental responsibility would be able to provide consent on their behalf and it would seem logical to involve that person in the procedure as much as is practicable. There is rarely a reason for a paramedic to be unable to document a complete set of vital signs measurements for any age of child and, regardless of age, a patient who is unable to give consent or is lacking in mental capacity must be treated according to their best interests. In summary, clinical holding is an appropriate technique to perform clinical assessment or urgently required interventions for a child or young person who is unable to give their consent. The use of clinical holding in paramedic practice should be supported by policy and guidance documents, and paramedic registrants should have appropriate training.

In contrast to clinical holding, restraint should be used only when it is necessary to give essential treatment or to prevent a child from significantly injuring themselves or others. Once a decision has been made that it is lawful and ethically acceptable to override a refusal of treatment, the appropriate use of force and/or restraint may be employed to provide that treatment. However, paramedics must look at the patient's overall interests and whether imposing treatment is a proportionate interference given the expected benefits. Where possible, the decision to use restraint should be made in consultation with a team (be that other professionals or senior colleagues who can provide advice).

Importantly, paramedics must consider if imposing treatment could damage the young person's current and future relationships with healthcare providers and undermine their trust in the medical profession. It is important for young people to understand that restraint of any form to provide treatment is used only as a last resort and not until other options for treatment have been explored. The child and the family must be offered continual support and information throughout the period of treatment.

If, after spending as much time as is practicable, it is impossible to persuade a child to co-operate with essential treatment, the clinician in charge of the patient's care may decide that restraint is appropriate. Members of the health team should be given an opportunity to express their views and to participate in the decision making, although ultimate responsibility rests with the clinician in charge of care. All staff require support and should not be asked to be involved in restraining a child without proper training.

Tips for Practice

The legislation concerning children and young people is complex and may not always provide the answer to your clinical scenario. Make sure you know how to access decision-making support in your area of practice.

Paramedics are likely to encounter children in emergency situations. If consent is not possible, do what is needed to stabilise the patient and act in their best interests. Legal guidance can be sought once emergency action has been taken.

Children and young people can be challenging to assess. They also may not appreciate how important it is for you to measure their vital signs. Use of distraction and clinical holding are appropriate techniques to enable effective assessment.

Summary

Paediatric law and ethics are complex, and support should always be sought when dealing with challenging cases that may involve decisions around consent, capacity or disagreement between parents and medical professionals. However, the law does provide very specific guidance to enable medical practitioners to undertake their role in delivering safe and effective healthcare to children and young people in a variety of circumstances. Despite being registered healthcare professionals, paramedics cannot be expected to have knowledge of each piece of legislation relating to the care of a child, but should know where to access this information and how to use it in the course of their clinical practice.

Recommended Reading

British Medical Association (2016) *Children and young people ethical toolkit*. Available at: www.bma.org.uk/advice/employment/ethics/children-and-young-people/ children-and-young-peoples-ethics-tool-kit/1-basic-principles.

General Medical Council (GMC) (2007) *0–18 Years: Guidance for All Doctors*. Available at: www .gmc-uk.org/-/media/documents/0_18_years_english_0418pdf_48903188.pdf.

General Medical Council (GMC) (2013) *Intimate Examinations and Chaperones*. Available at: www.gmc-uk.org/-/media/documents/maintaining-boundaries-intimate-examinations-and- chaperones_pdf-58835231.pdf.

References

British Medical Association (2016) *Children and young people ethical toolkit*. Available at: www.bma.org.uk/advice/employment/ethics/children-and-young-people/ children-and-young-peoples-ethics-tool-kit/1-basic-principles.

Children's Commissioner for England (2017) *Briefing: Children's Mental Healthcare in England*. Available at: www.childrenscommissioner.gov.uk/wp-content/uploads/2017/10/ Childrens-Commissioner-for-England-Mental-Health-Briefing-1.1.pdf.

College of Paramedics (2017) *Paramedic Curriculum Guidance*, 4th ed. Bridgwater: College of Paramedics.

Department of Health (2015). *The Mental Health Act 1983: Code of Practice*. Norwich: The Stationery Office.

General Medical Council (GMC) (2007) *0–18 Years: Guidance for All Doctors*. Available at: www .gmc-uk.org/-/media/documents/0_18_years_english_0418pdf_48903188.pdf.

General Medical Council (GMC) (2012) *Protecting Children and Young People*. Available at: www .gmc-uk.org/-/media/documents/Protecting_children_and_young_people___English_1015. pdf_48978248.pdf.

General Medical Council (GMC) (2013) *Intimate Examinations and Chaperones*. Available at: www.gmc-uk.org/-/media/documents/maintaining-boundaries-intimate-examinations-and- chaperones_pdf-58835231.pdf.

Guidelines and Audit Implementation Network (2011) *Guidelines on the Use of the Mental Health (Northern Ireland) Order 1986*. Available at: www.rqia.org.uk/RQIA/files/4e/4ee9f634-be47- 4398-afc9-906a20ff3198.pdf.

Medical Protection (2016) *Chaperones*. Available at: www.medicalprotection.org/uk/resources/ factsheets/england/england-factsheets/uk-chaperones.

Royal College of Nursing (2010) *Restrictive physical intervention and therapeutic holding for children and young people: Guidance for Nursing Staff*, 3rd ed. London: Royal College of Nursing.

Royal College of Nursing (2017) *Principles of Consent: Guidance for Nursing Staff*. London: Royal College of Nursing.

Statistics Portal (2018) *Child population (0–14) as a percentage of the total population in the United Kingdom (UK) from 2013 to 2060*. Available at: www.statista.com/statistics/478558/children-population-percentage-of-total-united-kingdom-uk.

Waller, L (2011) Ethics, law and paediatric medicine. *Journal of Paediatrics and Child Health*, 47: 620–23.

Wheeler, R (2006) *Gillick* or Fraser? A plea for consistency over competence in children: *Gillick* and Fraser are not interchangeable. *BMJ*, 332: 807.

UK Cases

A County Council v SB [2010] EWHC 2528 (Fam)

Attorney General's Reference (No 3 of 1994) [1997] 3 WLR 421

Bolam v Friern Hospital Management Committee [1957] 1 WLR 583

Bolitho v City & Hackney Health Authority [1997] 3 WLR 1151

Gillick v West Norfolk & Wisbech Area Health Authority [1986] UKHL 7

Glass v UK [2004] CFLQ 339

GMC v Bawa-Garba [2018] EWHC 76

Hart v Brown [1972] 289 A 2D 386

James and Evans v Alder Hey Children's NHS Foundation Trust [2018] EWHC 308 (Fam)

Paton v British Pregnancy Advisory Service [1978] 2 All ER 987

Paton v UK (1980) EHRR 408

R (Axon) v Secretary of State for Health [2006] EWCA 37

Re A (A Minor) (Wardship: Medical Treatment) [1993] 1 FLR 386

Re A (Children) (Conjoined Twins: Surgical Separation) [2001] Fam 147, CA

Re B (A Minor) (Wardship: Medical Treatment) [1990] 1 WLR 1421, CA

Re L (Medical Treatment: Gillick Competency) [1998] 2 FLR 819

Re R (A Minor) (Wardship: Consent to Treatment) [1992] Fam 11, CA

Re S (A Minor) (Consent to Medical Treatment) [1994] 2 FLR 1065

Re T (A Minor) (Wardship: Medical Treatment) [1997] 1 WLR 242, CA

Re W (A Minor) (Medical Treatment: Court Justification) [1993] Fam 64

Re Wyatt (A Child) (Medical Treatment: Continuation of Order) [2005] EWHC 693 (Fam)

St George's Healthcare Trust v S [1998] 3 All ER 673

Yates and Gard v Great Ormond Street Hospital for Children NHS Foundation Trust [2017] EWCA Civ 410; [2017] EWHC 1909 (Fam)

EU Cases

Vo v France [2004] 2 FCR 577, ECtHR

UK Legislation

Adults with Incapacity (Scotland) Act 2000

Age of Legal Capacity (Scotland) Act 1991

Age of Majority Act (Northern Ireland) 1969

Children Act 1989

Children's Act 2004

Children (Northern Ireland) Order 1995

Children (Scotland) Act 1995

Children Services Co-operation Act (Northern Ireland) 2015

Family Law Reform Act 1969

Human Rights Act 1998

Human Rights Act 2008

Human Tissue Act 2004

Law Reform (Parent and Child) (Scotland) Act 1986

Mental Capacity Act 2005

Mental Capacity (NI) Act 2016

Mental Health Act 1983

Mental Health (Scotland) Act 2015

Mental Health (Wales) Measure 2010

Mental Health (Northern Ireland) Order 1986

Chapter 12

Law and Ethics in Palliative Medicine and End-of-Life Care

Tom Mallinson

"You matter because you are you,
and you matter to the end of your life.
We will do all we can not only to help you die peacefully,
but also to live until you die."
Dame Cicely Saunders - Founder of Modern Palliative Medicine

Introduction

The specialty of palliative medicine concerns itself with the management of patients for whom the focus of care is symptom control and management. While many think of the Hospice movement founded by Dame Cicely Saunders when we consider palliative medicine (Richmond 2005; Twycross 2005), for a majority of patients receiving palliative and end-of-life care, this does not occur in a hospice setting (Pivodic et al. 2016). This care is likely to be multi-dimensional, taking into account social, psychological and spiritual factors as well as physiologic and medical issues. Palliative medicine is also a truly multi-professional field of medicine, which relies on the expertise not only of physicians, but also of specialist nurses, physiotherapists, occupational therapists, social workers and psychologists to make someone's last days truly matter. Paramedics are also increasingly becoming involved in end-of-life care decision making, either as part of their role in a primary care team or through frontline ambulance work (Pettifer and Bronnert 2013; Collen 2017; Kirk et al. 2017).

Increasingly, the terms 'palliative' and 'end-of-life care' are being used to encompass not only patients in the last hours or days of life, but more widely to include patients with any advanced and progressive disease, where there is an acknowledgement that medical management will not lead to a curative outcome. This will include conditions such as heart failure, chronic obstructive pulmonary disease and dementia.

There is a wide range of documentation which may be used in the management of palliative patients. Much of this documentation will discuss the patient's wishes in relation to their treatment and about decision making in the event that they are unable to make further decisions themselves. Some of this documentation will be legally binding, while some will contain advice, guidance and further information relating to the patient and their medical situation. Paramedics must be able to incorporate both sources of information into any management plan they are formulating for a patient who is reaching the end of their life.

Lasting Power of Attorney

England and Wales

A Lasting Power of Attorney (LPA) can be made by someone over the age of 18 and is chosen by the patient as someone who they want to be able to make decisions on their behalf when they lack capacity (*they are donating this ability*). There are two different types of LPA: LPA for health and welfare and LPA for property and financial affairs. This chapter will only cover LPA for health and welfare, also known as personal welfare (LPA-PW). These attorneys can make decisions when a person lacks capacity to make a specific welfare decision, although the person may put restrictions on the decisions that the LPA-PW can make (Office of the Public Guardian 2018).

In practice, if a patient has an LPA-PW, the attorney should be contacted, where practicable, to advise on any healthcare decision made for that patient. The decisions made by the attorney must still be guided by the principles of the Mental Capacity Act 2005 and the best interests test (section 4(a)). If there is more than one person appointed as LPA-PW, then the document may state whether they are to come to a decision together, whether they may make a decision independently or whether they must make some decisions together and may make others independently (section 10(4)). This means that they must work together on all matters, or *jointly* and *severally* where they can act together or separately as they subsequently choose. It could also be specified that the attorneys must act jointly for certain decisions; these may be specifically important or difficult decisions. Replacement attorneys can also be nominated in cases where an attorney dies or becomes incapacitated. If it is not stated on the document, the default presumption is that they must make decisions jointly (section 10(5)).

While an LPA gives the attorney the power to make decisions on behalf of the patient in relation to certain matters, the attorney must still make such decisions in the patient's *best interests*; this includes giving due consideration to the patient's beliefs and decisions prior to losing their capacity. The attorney must also register the LPA with the Public Guardian in order for it to be valid.

Northern Ireland

In Northern Ireland, the Mental Capacity Act (Northern Ireland) 2016 sets out a statutory provision for decision making on behalf of people who do not have capacity. Furthermore, the Enduring Power of Attorney (NI) Order 1987 makes provision for individuals with capacity to allow a second individual to have an Enduring Power of Attorney in relation to decisions made about their care if or when they lose capacity in the future. An Enduring Power of Attorney can give two forms of authority: a general authority and a specific authority. A general authority allows for any decisions to be made on behalf of the incapacitated individual, while a specific authority has restrictions or conditions applied.

Scotland

In Scotland, the Adults with Incapacity (Scotland) Act 2000 applies to those over the age of 16 who have capacity to appoint a welfare attorney to make decisions on their behalf once they lose the capacity to make these decisions for themselves. There is also provision in Scottish law for a Sheriff to appoint a welfare guardian for individuals who do not have capacity to choose their own welfare attorney (Scottish Government 2011).

Advance Directives

Advance Decisions to Refuse Treatment

Advance Decisions to Refuse Treatment (ADRTs) enable adults with capacity to refuse specific medical interventions for a time in the future when they lack capacity. In England and Wales, this is covered by the Mental Capacity Act 2005. In Northern Ireland, an ADRT is recognised under common law, and while there is currently no statutory *provision* for ADRTs, there is statutory *recognition* of them. More specifically, the Mental Capacity Act (Northern Ireland) 2016 requires that an advance decision should be complied with if it is valid and applicable under common law. There is a similar situation in Scotland, where the Adults with Incapacity (Scotland) Act 2000 instructs that account must be taken of the past wishes of an adult patient, but does not provide further statutory enforcement of such documents.

An ADRT *only* comes into effect when the person lacks capacity and the decision that is being made is the one to which the ADRT pertains. They are normally very specific, for example, refusing artificial ventilation or another specific type of life-sustaining treatment. Sometimes an ADRT may be particularly complex or there may be concerns about its contents or validity (Amblum-Almer 2016). If there is dispute or doubt about the validity of an ADRT in an emergency setting, then the paramedic should document why they are in doubt about the validity of the document and should continue to follow their normal best interests decision-making processes, and the receiving hospital should be made aware of the validity concerns as soon as is practicable.

Such a case may need to be referred to the Court of Protection. While the Court makes its determination, life-sustaining treatment, or treatment to prevent a serious deterioration in the patient's condition, may continue (Mental Capacity Act 2005).

Where a patient suffering a mental disorder has a valid ADRT, it may be appropriate to detain ('section') the patient in order to provide treatment under the powers of the Mental Health Act 1983. Further information about this is available in Chapter 9, which covers mental health law.

It is important to note that even if an ADRT is in place, this may be invalidated if the patient has elected another individual to hold an LPA (for personal welfare) and has given this individual the power to make the same decision as that documented in the ADRT. In this case, the decision-making ability relating to this issue has passed to the attorney and has therefore invalidated the ADRT. An ADRT is also invalid if it has been withdrawn and may be invalid if the patient has acted in a way which is clearly inconsistent with the ADRT (Mental Capacity Act 2005).

An ADRT can be both verbal and written; however, for life-sustaining treatment, it *must* meet the criteria set out by the Mental Capacity Act 2005 and be made by a capacitous person over the age of 18 in writing, be signed by the person making the decision (or by another person on that person's behalf) and also be signed by a witness. They do not need to be written with the input of a solicitor and they do not need to be documented in any formal way above what is set out in the Mental Capacity Act 2005. They may also be written in layman's terms. Once signed, they form a legally binding document and any person who knowingly treats a patient against the ADRT could be found guilty of the tort of battery.

There are a number of reasons why a healthcare professional may have reason to doubt whether an ADRT is valid (Amblum-Almer 2016). Core issues which may lead to questioning the validity of an ADRT may include whether the patient has done anything which clearly contradicts the ADRT, if the patient has directly withdrawn their decision or if the patient has subsequently conferred the power of attorney to another individual. If an ADRT specifically refuses life-sustaining treatment, it must be in writing. It can be written by someone other than the patient and can be recorded as a specific document or within the healthcare notes. It must be signed by the patient and also witnessed. The statement must also be clear that the decision made is still valid even if life is at risk.

If a healthcare professional concludes that the ADRT is not valid for a specific reason, it may still be taken into consideration as a prior expression of the patient's wishes at a point in the past, even if it does not have legal authority.

ReSPECT Forms

ReSPECT stands for Recommended Summary Plan for Emergency Care and Treatment. The ReSPECT initiative has been developed by a multi-disciplinary team, including representatives of various royal colleges, associations and patient groups (Fritz et al. 2017). The ReSPECT working group has developed a number of resources for patients to document their wishes for a future emergency where they lack the capacity to make a decision about their care at that time. The ReSPECT forms are designed to be an easy-to-access reference form providing a summary of the patient's wishes for advance decision making. They are designed to be kept with the patient at all times, for easy access and reference. It is likely that as ReSPECT forms are introduced across the UK, ambulance clinicians will be exposed to them more often and will be able to use their contents to inform the clinical decision-making process. It is important that ReSPECT is seen as a process that is not linked to end of life/palliative care only, but is seen as a natural conversation at any point during life. It is also not a replacement for a DNACPR form as it is not only about resuscitation from cardiac arrest. A number of people may have ReSPECT forms that state that he/she is for resuscitation and it is important that this distinction is highlighted so that the presence of a form does not lead to the assumption of no CPR.

DNACPR Forms

The terminology used in relation to forms indicating advance decisions against cardiopulmonary resuscitation is important and has evolved over recent years. Historically, the term 'Do Not Resuscitate' (DNR) was superseded by 'Do Not Attempt Resuscitation' (DNAR). However, the term 'resuscitation' is recognised as a broad term encompassing other forms of resuscitation such as intravenous fluid resuscitation; therefore, these terms have now largely been replaced by DNACPR decision documents. This makes it clear that the documents specifically and only apply to cardiopulmonary resuscitation. An example of a DNACPR form is in Appendix A.

There has also been a move away from referring to such documents as Orders, as they are intended to guide treatment decisions in a crisis situation. There is also the acknowledgement that a patient with a DNACPR in place (for example, for a progressive neurological disease) may still benefit from some degree of resuscitation in the case of cardiac or respiratory arrest due to a clearly reversible cause. To this end, it is better practice to refer to such documents as DNACPR decision documents. Paramedics are increasingly becoming involved in the care of patients with DNACPR forms in place and it is vital that they are confident incorporating DNACPR forms into their clinical practice (Armitage and Jones 2017). An example of a DNACPR form is included for reference in Appendix A. Regardless of visual differences, it is important such forms should be clear, concise and easily recognisable.

It is also important to recognise that, unlike an ADRT, a DNACPR decision document is not legally binding in the UK (Pitcher et al. 2017). The decision of whether or not to offer or initiate a specific clinical intervention (in this case cardiopulmonary resuscitation (CPR)) rests with the clinician responsible for the patient's care. Therefore, there may be occasions where the attending clinician makes the decision to undertake CPR when a DNACPR decision form is in place. In such a situation, the clinician would be expected to justify this decision in the same way as any other clinical decision. The two most common reasons for undertaking CPR in such situations would be if the respiratory or cardiac arrest was due to an unforeseen issue leading to circumstances not envisaged when the DNACPR form was completed, or if a DNACPR decision was temporarily suspended. An example of such a situation would be a patient with a progressive neurological disease and a tracheostomy. Such a patient may have a DNACPR in place to ensure that CPR was not undertaken in the case of disease progression leading to cardiac arrest. However, CPR may still be appropriate to resuscitate the individual from a blocked or dislodged tracheal tube. A DNACPR decision may also be suspended temporarily. This often occurs when the patient is undergoing a planned procedure, such as cardioversion, which carries the risk of inducing cardiac arrest, and where resuscitation would be immediately available. DNACPR decisions are also often suspended for patients undergoing general anaesthesia for surgery. Some DNACPR forms may also have specific instructions or a specific duration, after which they are no longer in effect.

✴ Case Study: DNACPR

You are working in an urban area on a single-crew response car for the ambulance service. You are called to the home of a 30-year-old man called Mr Jones; he is well known to you as you have attended to him on previous occasions when his carers have phoned 999. He suffered a diving accident some years ago which has left him quadriplegic and reliant on a ventilator. You are aware that he has a DNACPR form in place and that a copy is kept in a folder by his bed. You have seen this form recently and know it is filled out appropriately and has not expired.

This form was completed after Mr Jones experienced a respiratory arrest secondary to pneumonia and was admitted to hospital for a prolonged period of time and required Level 3 (Intensive Care) support. After this episode, he decided he did not want to experience that again and put a DNACPR in place in case he experienced another respiratory arrest due to pneumonia. He does not have any other advance decision documented and has not appointed a power of attorney.

Today his carers have called because he has suffered a respiratory arrest due to mechanical failure of his ventilator. On your arrival, one carer is ventilating him with a self-inflating ambu-bag using room air via his tracheostomy tube. Good air entry is being achieved and his chest sounds clear with equal air entry and no added sounds. He has a weak irregular radial pulse. His vital signs are: SpO_2 93%, HR 40–60 irregular with multiple ectopics, BP 82/34 mmHg. Capillary refill is 3 seconds centrally but 6 seconds peripherally.

You suspect Mr Jones is peri-arrest due to a period of apnoea and subsequent hypoxaemia. You find his DNACPR and note that it is still valid and in date. The form indicates that 'CPR could be successful but the likely outcome would not be of overall benefit to the patient. The patient does not want CPR to be attempted'. The form is signed by Mr Jones' GP, his specialist nurse and his mother. The form indicates that all three witnessed Mr Jones express this opinion.

As you finish reviewing the DNACPR form, your monitor alerts you that Mr Jones' heart rate is dropping significantly and is now between 30 and 40 beats per minute with a blood pressure of 75/30.

What is the Best Course of Action Here?

At this stage, Mr Jones is not in cardiac arrest and therefore the DNACPR is not applicable; consequently, Mr Jones could have his airway suctioned and be ventilated with 100% oxygen. Furthermore, you could gain intravascular access and administer atropine to correct his heart rate and inotropes or vasopressors to improve his blood pressure if this is within your skill set.

If he went into cardiac arrest now, two options are open to you: acknowledge the DNACPR form and do not commence resuscitation; or while acknowledging that a DNACPR form is in place, you could consider that the cause of this arrest was unforeseen at the time of completing the DNACPR form and therefore it is not applicable in this situation, and thus undertake resuscitation. As discussed above, a DNACPR form is not legally binding, but does provide information about the patient's prior wishes. In this case, the clinician must be able to defend their decision, whether they choose to withhold or commence CPR. The defence for undertaking CPR in this case would be that the mechanical fault with the ventilator was an unanticipated occurrence which was not envisaged when the DNACPR form was completed.

What would you do in this situation?

Ethical Considerations

Whilst the classical ethical principles underpinning healthcare ethics are usually stated as being non-maleficence (causing no harm), beneficence (causing benefit), respect for the patient's autonomy and justice (utility or fairness in a wider sense) (Parkinson 2015), an outline of the different ethical positions is given in Chapter 3.

However, these four overarching principles can be directly applied and may be a helpful aid to decision making, particularly in end-of-life care. An example could be as follows: a patient reaching the end of their life due to chronic obstructive pulmonary disease (COPD) is in the last days of life and is semi-conscious. The family have called 999 and have requested that the attending paramedic provide intravenous fluid therapy to the patient. In deciding whether this is an ethical intervention, the paramedic could first consider if the parenteral fluids could cause harm to the patient (non-maleficence), if they would benefit the patient (beneficence) and whether providing this intervention respects the patient's autonomy, before, finally, considering if providing this intervention to this patient is fair and just.

In terms of non-maleficence, there is a harm involved here. Actual and possible harm is associated with this intervention: there is the direct harm associated with a needle piercing skin and a blood vessel; the risk of unintended injury from this needle; and there may also be other harms that are less clearly foreseeable, both physical and psychological. In terms of beneficence, it is unclear if intravenous fluids would benefit this patient through improving symptoms or extending life; however, it may be that this patient is semi-conscious due to an easily reversible cause, which could be addressed with intravenous fluids. When considering this intervention in relation to respect for the patient's autonomy, the paramedic would need to know what the patient's stated wishes had been before they lost the capacity for decision making, and advance directives and documents such as the ReSPECT form could be helpful in this regard (Resuscitation Council UK 2018).

While these four principles are the basis for all healthcare ethics, there are a number of other core concepts which are central to healthcare ethics in relation to end-of-life and palliative medicine. These concepts can directly or indirectly influence the decision-making process of a paramedic attending a patient with palliative care needs.

🚑 Case Study: Patient-Centred vs Utilitarian

You are working on a single-crewed vehicle in a rural area. You are called in the early hours of the morning to a patient you know well, a 62-year-old woman who has end-stage COPD. She had phoned 999, but was unable to speak due to breathlessness. On your arrival, she is breathless and distressed; she has a DNACPR document and an advance care plan, which details her refusal to be conveyed to hospital. She has palliative medications prescribed and available at home. After you administer two doses of subcutaneous morphine, the patient's breathing improves, but she is still upset and does not want to be left alone.

You have arranged the out-of-hours palliative care specialist nurse to attend, but they will take at least 40 minutes to arrive. You feel the patient is likely to die within hours. You are aware that multiple high-priority calls are being held in your area and the next nearest resource is at least an hour away.

What Would You Decide to Do in This Situation?

The patient is requesting you stay and provide reassurance, although no further medical input is currently required. The patient does not want to be conveyed to hospital and a specialist is en route. In terms of providing patient-centred care, you should not leave this patient until they are either less distressed or someone else arrives to comfort them. Many clinicians would also argue strongly that this patient should not die alone and would feel uneasy about leaving her alone at home. However, taking a wider utilitarian stance, it could be argued that in terms of upholding beneficence and justice at a societal level, your time and skills would be best used by attending to another emergency call and leaving this patient alone at home. This is a difficult situation and one where a clinician's duty of care to their patient is to some extent in conflict with their wider duty of care to society, and certainly their employer's duty of care to a larger population.

The Principle of Double Effect

A core ethical consideration for paramedics providing treatments to patients nearing the end of their life is the principle of double effect (Billings 2011; Shaw 2002). This is where it is accepted that a specific treatment given for one desired effect may also cause a second, less desirable effect. The most common example of this is giving a strong analgesic in the knowledge that it will depress cardiorespiratory function and shorten someone's life. Such an action is deemed to be morally, and likely legally, acceptable when such an action adheres to three rules: first, this is only acceptable for a patient who is already dying; second, the intervention must be *right and proper* professional practice; and, third, the motive for such an intervention must be to improve symptoms and not to shorten life.

One could of course argue against any of these three rules. For example, a consequentialist ethicist may argue that the morality of any act is dependent on the outcome caused, and therefore even if your motive was to improve symptom burden (as in rule three), if your action also caused a patient's life to end prematurely, this could be judged to be an immoral act, as it resulted in an early death. It could also be argued that someone's motive for an action does not change whether such an action is intrinsically right or wrong, making rule three unhelpful.

> ***Pause for Thought: The Sulmasy Test***
>
> *Dr Sulmasy (1996) has posited a test to allow doctors (and indeed paramedics) to check what their intention really is. The clinician should ask themselves: 'If the patient were not to die after my actions, would I feel that I had failed to accomplish what I had set out to do?'*

Euthanasia

Euthanasia, the act of actively ending someone's life, is not legal in the UK (NHS Choices 2017; Royal College of Nurses 2016), although support for euthanasia is growing (Danyliv and O'Neill 2015). An ethical argument to legalise euthanasia could be based on the principle of autonomy, arguing that an individual should have the autonomy to choose the time and manner of their death. The counter-arguments are legion, one of the core opposing positions being the principle of the sanctity of life, which states that all human life is sacred and intrinsically special. This argument is closely aligned with some religious philosophies and is also often used to argue against contraception and abortion. Another argument is that euthanasia places value on people's lives and therefore assigns a lesser value to some lives (the sick or disabled) than others. It has also been argued that once legalised, euthanasia would create a slippery slope, leading to involuntary or coercive euthanasia. A more practical argument is that with advances in modern palliative care, euthanasia should not be needed, as symptoms can be controlled fully, allowing people to be comfortable in the time leading up to their death.

There is, unfortunately, also often confusion about what is and is not euthanasia. It is important as a clinician to be clear as to what acts or omissions are not euthanasia. The act of sedation at the end of life to control distressing symptoms is not euthanasia, nor is the discontinuation of life prolonging interventions (e.g. parenteral nutrition, hydration or ventilation) where such interventions are futile. Issuing a DNACPR, terminating resuscitation or not starting resuscitation where it would be futile are also not forms of euthanasia.

The Acts/Omissions Doctrine

This doctrine determines the ethical difference of whether a person actively intervenes to bring about a result, or omits to act in circumstances in which it can be foreseen that as an outcome of the omission, the same result occurs.

This doctrine is most often applied to euthanasia. Suppose someone wishes another person dead. If they bring about this other person's death, they are a murderer. But if they discover this person is in danger of death and fail to act to save them, they are not acting and therefore, according to the doctrine, are not a murderer. 'Doing nothing' can be a way of 'doing something'. The absence of bodily movement can also constitute acting deliberately, and depending on the context may be an act of negligence through deceiving, betraying or killing. Nevertheless, criminal law often finds it convenient to distinguish discontinuing an intervention, which

> **Pause for Thought**
>
> The trolley problem was highlighted in Chapter 3 and is an example of the acts/omissions doctrine. The situation is structurally similar to others in which utilitarian reasoning seems to lead to one course of action, but a person's values or principles may oppose it. Some hold that there is no morally significant difference between the two; therefore, occasions may arise when killing a person may be no less bad or wrong than letting the person die.

is permissible, from bringing about a result, which may not be if, for instance, the result is the death of a patient. The question is whether the difference (if there is one) between acting and omitting to act can be described or defined in a way that bears any moral weight.

✳ Case Study: Breathlessness

You are undertaking a home visit to a 60-year-old man with breathing difficulties. On arrival, the patient is in severe respiratory distress and is centrally cyanosed. He is cachexic and looks exhausted; he gestures to a letter by his bed detailing a diagnosis of widespread metastatic carcinoma made a year ago. He manages to tell you that he doesn't want to go to hospital and just wants to die at home. He asks you to stop his suffering and end his life.

Legally, euthanasia and assisted suicide are illegal in the UK, so you cannot actively end his life. It is of course still legal to treat him by providing symptomatic relief. However, taking him to hospital would be against his wishes and therefore inappropriate. If treatment were to be provided to ease his breathlessness, for example through the use of opiates, it may be that this treatment may also shorten his life. This may be acceptable as a result of the principle of double effect if the three rules of this principle are met, as discussed previously. This man does not appear to have made an advance directive and there is no DNACPR form. There is also no indication that he has a power of attorney arrangement in place.

How would you treat this man's breathlessness?

How would you feel if he stopped breathing soon after you had administered treatment for his breathlessness?

What would you do if this patient went into cardiac arrest?

From this case study, it appears that this patient would benefit from treatment aimed at improving his symptoms. Currently, morphine is the most widely available appropriate drug that can be carried by paramedics for this indication. Oxygen therapy may also be considered and may improve symptoms in patients where hyperaemia is a problem – most commonly, a target oxygen saturation of 88–90% is utilised. In a case such as this, although opiate doses will usually be started low and subsequently increased, it may be the case that an initial dose will lead to significant respiratory depression, hypercapnia and possibly apnoea. If so, this would be a clear example of the principle of double effect, where the intention was to improve symptoms and an unwanted effect was to hasten death. It is important to fully understand this concept to ensure that you are practising appropriately, but also for your own peace of mind in such situations. If this patient were to suffer a cardiac arrest, it would most likely be inappropriate to commence resuscitation. This patient has a clear history of a progressive, terminal illness and it is unlikely that a resuscitation attempt would be successful or appropriate.

Summary

The current law surrounding death and dying in the UK is complex and ever-changing. It is important for paramedics to have a good grounding in the concepts involved and also to know how to stay up to date with new developments. The same can be said for the ethical concepts involved in end-of-life decision making. Although some ethical principles have stood the test of time, there are constantly discussions and developments in the field of medical ethics. It has been said that a health service can be judged by the quality of the end-of-life care it provides. A similar assertion could be made about paramedic practice, for although palliative care is only a small element of a paramedic's scope of practice, it is an important one and is an area in which there is little room for substandard care. We must strive to provide the highest quality of care to our patients, and help them live life to the full until they die.

Recommended Reading

Ashcroft, RE et al. (eds) (2007) *Principles of Health Care Ethics*, 2nd ed. Chichester: Wiley-Blackwell.

Brazier, M and Cave, E (2016) *Medicine, Patients and the Law*, 6th ed. Oxford: Oxford University Press.

Randall, F and Downie, RS (2002) *Palliative Care Ethics: A Companion for All Specialities*, 2nd ed. Oxford: Oxford University Press.

Watson, M et al. (2005). *Oxford Handbook of Palliative Care*, 2nd ed. Oxford: Oxford Medical Publications.

References

Amblum-Almer, J (2016) Critical evaluation of advance statements from patients lacking mental capacity. *Journal of Paramedic Practice*, 8(9): 463–69.

Armitage, E and Jones, C (2017) Paramedic attitudes towards DNACPR orders. *Journal of Paramedic Practice*, 9(10): 445–52.

Billings, JA (2011) Double effect: a useful rule that alone cannot justify hastening death. *Journal of Medical Ethics*, 37(7): 437–40.

Collen, A (2017). *Decision Making in Paramedic Practice*. Bridgwater: Class Professional Publishing.

Danyliv, A and O'Neill, C (2015) Attitudes towards legalising physician provided euthanasia in Britain: the role of religion over time. *Social Science & Medicine*, 128: 52–56.

Foot, P (1967) The problem of abortion and the doctrine of the double effect. *Oxford Review*, 5: 1–7.

Fritz, Z, Slowther, A-M and Perkins, GD (2017) Resuscitation policy should focus on the patient not the decision. *BMJ*, 356: j813.

Kirk, A et al. (2017) Paramedics and their role in end-of-life care: perceptions and confidence. *Journal of Paramedic Practice*, 9(2): 71–79.

NHS Choices (2017) *Euthanasia and assisted suicide*. Available at: www.nhs.uk/conditions/euthanasia-and-assisted-suicide.

Office of the Public Guardian (2018) *LPA for financial decisions: make and register (complete pack)*. Available at: www.gov.uk/government/publications/make-a-lasting-power-of-attorney.

Parkinson, M (2015) Pain: highlighting the law and ethics of pain relief in end-of-life patients. *Journal of Paramedic Practice*, 7(7): 344–49.

Pettifer, A and Bronnert, R (2013). End of life care in the community: the role of ambulance clinicians. *Journal of Paramedic Practice*, 5(7): 394–99.

Pitcher, D et al. (2017). Emergency care and resuscitation plans. *BMJ*, 356: j876.

Pivodic, L et al. (2016) Place of death in the population dying from diseases indicative of palliative care need: a cross-national population-level study in 14 countries. *Journal of Epidemiology and Community Health*, 70(1):17-24.

Resuscitation Council UK (2015) *DNACPR model form* (adult). Available at: www.resus.org.uk/dnacpr/do-not-attempt-cpr-model-forms/.

Resuscitation Council UK (2018) *Recommended Summary Plan for Emergency Care and Treatment*. Available at: www.respectprocess.org.uk.

Richmond, C (2015) *Dame Cicely Saunders, founder of the modern hospice movement, dies. BMJ.* Available at: www.bmj.com/content/suppl/2005/07/18/331.7509.DC1.

Royal College of Nurses (2016) *When Someone Asks for Your Assistance to Die*, 2nd ed. London: Royal College of Nurses.

Scottish Government (2011) *Adults with Incapacity (Scotland Act) 2000: Code of Practice: For Persons Authorised under Intervention Orders and Guardians*. Edinburgh: Scottish Government.

Shaw, A (2002) Two challenges to the double effect doctrine: euthanasia and abortion. *Journal of Medical Ethics*, 28(2): 102–4.

Sulmasy, D (1996) The use and abuse of the principle of double effect. *Clinical Pulmonary Medicine*, 3(2): 86–90.

Twycross, R (2005) *A Tribute to Dame Cicely.* Available at: www.stchristophers.org.uk/about/damecicelysaunders/tributes

UK Legislation

Adult Support and Protection (Scotland) Act 2007

Adults with Incapacity (Scotland) Act 2000

Enduring Power of Attorney (NI) Order 1987

Mental Capacity Act 2005

Mental Capacity Act (Northern Ireland) 2016

Mental Health Act 1983

Mental Health (Care and Treatment) (Scotland) Act 2003

Appendix A: DNACPR model form (adult)

DO NOT ATTEMPT CARDIOPULMONARY RESUSCITATION

Adults aged 16 years and over   DNACPRadult.1(2015)

Name _____

Address _____

Date of birth _____

NHS number _____

Date of DNACPR decision:

/   /

DO NOT PHOTOCOPY

In the event of cardiac or respiratory arrest no attempts at cardiopulmonary resuscitation (CPR) are intended. All other appropriate treatment and care will be provided.

1	**Does the patient have capacity to make and communicate decisions about CPR?**	YES / NO

If "YES" go to box 2

If "NO", are you aware of a valid advance decision refusing CPR which is relevant to the current condition?"   If "YES" go to box 6 | YES / NO |

If "NO", has the patient appointed a Welfare Attorney to make decisions on their behalf? | YES / NO |
If "YES" they must be consulted.

All other decisions must be made in the patient's best interests and comply with current law.
Go to box 2

2	**Summary of the main clinical problems and reasons why CPR would be inappropriate, unsuccessful or not in the patient's best interests:**

3	**Summary of communication with patient (or Welfare Attorney). If this decision has not been discussed with the patient or Welfare Attorney state the reason why:**

4	**Summary of communication with patient's relatives or friends:**

5	**Names of members of multidisciplinary team contributing to this decision:**

6	**Healthcare professional recording this DNACPR decision:**

Name _____   Position _____

Signature _____   Date _____   Time _____

7	**Review and endorsement by most senior health professional:**

Signature _____   Name _____   Date _____

Review date (if appropriate): _____

Signature _____   Name _____   Date _____

Signature _____   Name _____   Date _____

Resuscitation Council UK, 2015.

Chapter 13

A Note on Uncontrolled Donation after Circulatory Death

Edd Bartlett

Introduction

This short chapter outlines the legal principles surrounding organ donation. This subject is perhaps not widely associated with paramedics, despite the fact that the profession is synonymous with the provision of out-of-hospital advanced life support. It is surprising that since only 25.8% of patients who have an out-of-hospital cardiac arrest in England are likely to achieve return of spontaneous circulation (Hawkes et al. 2017), more emphasis is not placed on considering the importance of organ donation. This chapter serves as an introduction to the topic and asks the reader to consider their viewpoint on the role of organ donation, and whether the paramedic profession may have more involvement in such decisions as the law surrounding this subject continues to evolve.

Background

In 2015/16, nearly 500 people on the transplant list died waiting for transplants (NHS Blood and Transplant 2017). The Organ Donation Taskforce was set up in 2006 to identify barriers to donation. One barrier they explored was the UK's position on non-heart beating donors. Non-heart beating donors have died following a cardiac arrest and are known as Donation after Circulatory Death donors (DCD donors). The Taskforce noted a perceived lack of legal clarity amongst clinicians on when they could continue treatment to preserve organs when that treatment was not in their patient's best interests medically and would normally be withdrawn (Organ Donation Taskforce 2008a).

Since this report, the legal position has been clarified and there has been an expansion of DCD programmes, and the number of donors has increased by over 50% (Academy of Medical Royal Colleges 2008; Department of Health 2009; NHS Blood and Transplant 2013). This has resulted in the Taskforce's target of a 50% increase in donor rates being achieved 'almost exclusively due to expansion of DCD programmes' (NHS Blood and Transplant 2013).

Categorisation for Organ Donors

Following the success of the increase in DCD programmes, NHS Blood and Transplant's strategy for 2020 looks at the potential for Maastricht Category I/II DCD being introduced across the UK following a pilot programme in Scotland (NHS Blood and Transplant 2013). The different Maastricht categories are outlined below.

Maastricht Categories	
Maastricht I	Organs are retrieved following an unexpected cardiac arrest outside of hospital.
Maastricht II	Organs are retrieved following an unexpected cardiac arrest in hospital.
Maastricht III	Organs are retrieved following an expected cardiac arrest following withdrawal of treatment.
Maastricht IV	Organs are retrieved following an expected cardiac arrest in a brainstem dead patient.

Pilot Models in the UK

Historically in the UK, organs have only been procured from Maastricht Category III and IV donors. The first hospital in the UK to introduce uncontrolled donation after cardiac death (uDCD) procedure was the Royal Infirmary of Edinburgh (Reed and Lua 2013), which ran a pilot in the Lothian region to explore the efficacy of introducing a uDCD procedure for patients who had an out-of-hospital cardiac arrest, or who had an untreatable cardiac arrest in the Emergency Department (ED). When treatment was considered futile chest compressions and ventilations continued to allow for organ donation to take place, subject to inclusion and exclusion criteria (Reed and Lua 2013).

In the Lothian procedure, once futility has been decided by the ED consultant and a second senior doctor, confirmation of registration in the Organ Donor Register, or another indication of wishes to donate, is established by a Specialist Nurse-Organ Donation. The patient's next of kin must also be available for consultation (Reed and Lua 2015, pp. 3, 6). If it is established that the patient is a potential donor, resuscitation continues while the family is consulted. This does not differ from the common practice of informing the family of futility in a normal ED resuscitation (Reed and Lua 2015, pp. 3, 6). Following consultation with the family and their authorisation, mechanical resuscitation continues to be used to preserve the organs until the transplant team is ready; only then is death formally pronounced (Reed and Lua 2015).

The Lothian procedure warrants praise for its thoroughness and transparency: its operation is underpinned by fundamental principles which emphasise a 'complete separation of resuscitation and consideration of organ donation' (Currie et al. 2014). This is strongly emphasised throughout the procedure document (Reed and Lua 2015). The only component of the procedure that could be considered to be at odds with Department of Health guidance and that could cause problems if it were to be applied in England and Wales (as the Department of Health guidance only applies in England and Wales) is 'continued resuscitation' (Department of Health 2009).

However, the guidance from the Department of Health appears not to take into consideration that the resuscitation — which is being taken to predominantly refer to external cardiac massage — is not being instigated, but continued, with continuing mechanical ventilation being considered acceptable (Department of Health 2009). As discussed above, it is commonplace for external cardiac massage to be continued while the family is informed that the resuscitation has been deemed futile in both in-hospital and out-of-hospital cardiac arrest. Sometimes resuscitation is also provided where doctors believe there to be no clinical benefit because the family continue to want it (Troug 2010).

There is no indication that continued external cardiac massage causes the patient any harm, provided that the family is consulted and, in the event of distress or objection, external cardiac massage is not continued. There is no reason to believe that extending the duration of external cardiac massage using a mechanical chest compression device to fulfil a person's desire to be an organ donor is not acceptable (Ave et al. 2016).

In other countries such as France and Spain, and in New York, USA, organs are also procured from patients who suffer an out-of-hospital cardiac arrest (Jox et al. 2016). While some of these countries, like France and Spain, have seen an increase in organ procurement following the introduction of uncontrolled Donation after Circulatory Death (uDCD), there are significant ethical concerns about the blurring of boundaries between active resuscitation and organ retrieval, and the potential for deceitful practices (Farrell et al. 2011; Jox et al. 2016).

The French-Spanish Model

In France and Spain, organs are procured from patients who have suffered an out-of-hospital cardiac arrest. The method of retrieving organs requires the use of a mechanical chest compression device to facilitate perfusion en route to the hospital after resuscitation has been deemed futile by the attending emergency medical services (Fondevila et al. 2012; Punch and Anderson 2012). In the French-Spanish model, it is only upon arrival at the hospital that the mechanical chest compression device is paused for at least five minutes so that death can be declared, despite a physician who could declare death being available on the response vehicle (Fondevila et al. 2012).

This delay in declaration of death has been criticised as a strategic decision to circumvent informing the next of kin that the person is being taken to hospital purely as a potential organ donor (Jox et al. 2016). There are also concerns about resource allocation, with an emergency response vehicle being 'tied up' with a person who doesn't require further medical assistance and might not even be accepted by the receiving organ retrieval team (Jox et al. 2016).

There have been a number of cases in France and Spain where patients destined for organ donation have developed restoration of spontaneous circulation. In some rare cases, neurological function has also been restored, with one person being discharged from hospital neurologically intact (Rodriguez-Arias et al. 2013; Jox et al. 2016). Mateos-Rodriguez et al. have responded to this by simply stating that: 'If these individuals had not been included in the protocol, resuscitation would have stopped after 30 min and the patients would not have survived' (2010, p. 906). This suggests that being a potential organ donor in France and Spain may be in a patient's best interests as it could slightly increase their chance of survival, although it also raises concerns about their resuscitation protocols and that they may be prematurely deeming resuscitation attempts futile. As death is declared at hospital, the patient doesn't 'come back' from a legally declared death, and Mateos-Rodriguez et al. make assurances that 'guidance for diagnosing death is strictly followed on arrival at the transplant centres' (Mateos-Rodriguez et al. 2010, p. 906).

A significant criticism of the French-Spanish uDCD model is the absence of transparency. In Spain, uDCD was practised for four years before it was explicitly authorised by the law (Jox et al. 2016). Both the French and Spanish laws were passed (in 2006 and 2000 respectively) without any stakeholder or public involvement. In contrast, the New York model actively involved key stakeholders in the development of its protocol (Jox et al. 2016).

Some authors raise concerns that in the French-Spanish models, there is Third World resuscitation and First World organ donation (Jox et al. 2016). If the introduction of uDCD was interpreted in this way in England and Wales, it could have catastrophic implications for public trust in organ donation. It is recommended by Reed and Lua (2013) that uDCD in the ED is carefully reviewed, as unconventional resuscitation interventions such as extracorporeal membrane oxygenation (ECMO) and coronary angiography become common practice. Should these interventions be considered potentially beneficial, it is recommended that it is ensured that patients are given the opportunity to benefit from these interventions, where appropriate, before donation is considered.

> **Pause for Thought**
>
> *Have you expressed your wishes for your organs after death?*

Consent Models

There are two main consent models used in the UK concerning organ donation: an 'opt-in' model and an 'opt-out' model. The opt-in model is widely recognised as an individual placing their name on the Organ Donor Register, although relatives can also give consent on the deceased's behalf if they are not on the Register.

In 2015, Wales introduced the UK's first 'opt-out' model, coined as a 'deemed consent' model as opposed to the term 'presumed consent' used in other European jurisdictions. Wales made the decision to introduce deemed consent following a public consultation which concluded that there was a public preference for a soft opt-out system. Such a system has been advocated by the British Medical Association (BMA) for some time, despite the Organ Donation Taskforce (ODT) concluding in 2008 that an opt-out system would not deliver a significant increase in organs (BMA 2017; ODT 2008b).

A common misconception is that the success of the Spanish system, with the highest rate of organ donation from deceased donors in the world (34.4 donors per million of the population in 2009), is due to presumed consent legislation. In fact, presumed consent was introduced in 1979, but donation rates only began to rise in 1989 following the introduction of the Organización Nacional de Transplantes (National Transplant Organization), which put a national network of dedicated clinicians in charge of the donation process (Farrell et al. 2011).

Legislation has now been passed by the UK parliament to introduce an opt-out system for England. The successful Organ Donation (deemed consent) Bill now awaits Royal assent to become law. It is expected that England will have this system in place by 2020 (NHS Blood and Transplant 2019). The Scottish Parliament are considering introducing similar legislation (British Medical Association 2019), whilst Northern Ireland continues to use an opt-out system. This would mean that family and friends can prevent organs from being procured if they believe the deceased did not wish to donate their organs (Human Tissue Authority 2014 (updated 2017), para 28). In the UK, which has one of the highest family refusal rates in the Western world and over 40% of families not consenting to donation, it is not guaranteed that moving to a soft opt-out system would result in an increase in organ procurement (NHS Blood and Transplant 2013).

Ethical Consideration within uDCD

Opt-out models have also been criticised as a breach of autonomy. With the rest of medicine moving away from paternalism and promoting patient autonomy, introducing an opt-out policy for donation is considered by some to be wrong. Veatch and Ross (2015) argue that under such as system, people's wishes will not be respected 25% of the time, and in some cultures this rate would be higher. On the other hand, the Organ Donation Taskforce (2008b, p. 8) described presumed consent as 'consent for the disorganised', perceiving its purpose as being to provide consent for those who had not found the time to register their consent. One of the key questions in the debate about these models is do opt-out models promote or violate autonomy?

Some writers go a step further, suggesting that a system of organ conscription should be introduced, often comparing it to the compulsory coronial autopsy (Jox et al. 2016). Harris (1992), a utilitarian philosopher, believes that informed consent and personal autonomy cannot be absolute rights; the reduction of suffering and saving the most lives possible must be the highest priorities. In such a system, there would be no option to opt out or for the wishes of relatives stating that their loved one did not want to be a donor to be respected.

> ### *Pause for thought*
>
> *Indeed it seems clear that the benefits from cadaver transplants are so great, and the reasons for objecting so transparently selfish or superstitious, that we should remove altogether the habit of seeking the consent of either the deceased or relatives. This we already do when post-mortem examinations are ordered without any consents being required and despite the fact that these too involve interference with the dignity of a dead body and the removal (albeit temporarily) of organs. It has always seemed to me curious that the state can order a post-mortem examination to satisfy its curiosity about the cause of death, but not order cadaver transplants in order to save the lives of living citizens.*
>
> **Harris (1992, pp. 102–3) in *Wonderwoman and Superman***

The procurement of organs from people who have suffered an out-of-hospital cardiac arrest is presumed to only be practical in an opt-out system. However, with advancements in information sharing and more ambulance trusts moving towards electronic patient records, it may soon be possible to share people's donation wishes in the same way that their resuscitation status and other care plans are now shared in some trusts.

Should uDCD Be Introduced Across the UK?

Before uDCD can be introduced across the whole of the UK, the relevant Departments of Health would have to produce a new position statement on continuing resuscitation to facilitate uDCD. Following this, uDCD could initially be introduced in appropriate emergency departments; once successfully established, a pilot uDCD protocol could be introduced in an urban environment where there are good ambulance response times and paramedics are available to provide clinical leadership at cardiac arrests where the decision to convey a potential donor is made.

Explicit opt-in consent is preferable for uDCD due to the invasive interventions required to preserve the organs. Also, due to the already traumatic nature of an out-of-hospital cardiac arrest, if the next of kin object to organ-preserving measures, clinicians should not proceed and recognition of life extinct should be confirmed on scene. If the patient is to be conveyed as a potential donor, it would be considered good practice for the ambulance crew to speak to a Specialist Nurse-Organ Donation prior to conveyance to ensure that the patient is suitable to be a donor. If this is not the case, conveyance would not be in the patient's best interests.

Clinicians having access to a patient's donation wishes have also seen concerns raised that this might compromise their duty of care, causing patients to be disadvantaged by premature cessation of resuscitation and the implementation of organ-preserving measures. However, the UK Donation Ethics Committee (2011, p. 20) has considered these concerns to be misplaced.

Ultimately, the efficacy of such a protocol is likely to influence its future, although the conveyance of a patient to the ED will mean that an ambulance is not available to respond to 999 calls for that period. If the project yielded more organs for transplant, the cost savings (for dialysis and other treatments given to those with organ failure) and lives saved may mitigate resourcing concerns.

Summary

The concept of uDCD is likely to be a new one to the reader. Whilst there are as yet no UK-wide models considering procedures associated with out-of-hospital cardiac arrest and uDCD, it is likely these will emerge as the legislation for organ donation changes in England, Northern Ireland and Wales. It is important to be mindful that uDCD protocols carry a hefty legal and ethical obligation, and it is paramount that they are undertaken in a legally and ethically satisfactory way. Not only will this ensure that the paramedic acts within the legal boundaries of their profession, but it will ensure that the risk of public backlash is significantly decreased and that there will be an increase in the number of kidneys and livers available for transplantation in the UK.

Recommended Reading

Jox, R, Assadi, G and Marckmann, G (eds) (2016) *Organ Transplantation in Times of Donor Shortage Challenges and Solutions.* London: Springer.

Reed, M and Lua, S (2013) Uncontrolled organ donation after circulatory death: potential donors in the emergency department. *Emergency Medical Journal*, 31(9): 741–44.

References

Academy of Medical Royal Colleges (2008) *A Code of Practice for the Diagnosis and Confirmation of Death.* London: PPG Design and Print Ltd.

Ave A, Shaw, D and Gardiner D (2016) Cardiopulmonary resuscitation of brain-dead organ donors: a literature review and suggestions for practice. *Transplant International* 29(1): 12–19.

British Medical Association (2017) *Organ Donation* (28 February 2017). Available at: www.bma.org.uk/collective-voice/policy-and-research/ethics/organ-donation, (accessed: 09 July 2017)

British Medical Association (2019) Organ donation in Scotland (26 February 2019) Available at: https://www.bma.org.uk/collective-voice/policy-and-research/ethics/organ-donation/scotland (accessed: 06 March 2019)

Currie, I et al. (2014) *The Royal Infirmary of Edinburgh Organ Donation from the Emergency Department Category II DCD Pilot Program.* Unpublished.

Department of Health (2009) *Legal issues relevant to non-heartbeating organ donation.* Department of Health.

Farrell, A, Price, D and Quigley, M (eds) (2011) *Organ Shortage Ethics, Law and Pragmatism.* Cambridge: Cambridge University Press.

Fondevila, C et al. (2012) Applicability and results of Maastricht Type 2 Donation after cardiac death liver transplantation. *American Journal of Transplantation*, 12(1): 162–70.

Harris J (1992) *Wonderwoman and Superman: Ethics of Human Biotechnology.* Oxford: Oxford University Press

Hawkes, C et al. (2017) Epidemiology and outcomes from out-of-hospital cardiac arrests in England. *Resuscitation*, 110: 133–40.

Human Tissue Authority (2014, updated 2017) *Code of Practice on the Human Transplantation (Wales) Act 2013*. Human Tissue Authority.

Jox, R, Assadi, G and Marckmann, G (eds) (2016) *Organ Transplantation in Times of Donor Shortage: Challenges and Solutions*. London: Springer.

Mateos-Rodriguez, A et al. (2010) Kidney transplant function using organs from non-heart-beating donors maintained by mechanical chest compressions. *Resuscitation*, 81(7): 904–7.

NHS Blood and Transplant (2013) *Taking Organ Transplantation to 2020: A Detailed Strategy*. London: Department of Health.

NHS Blood and Transplant (2017) *Organ Donation and Transplantation Activity Report 2016/17*. London: Department of Health.

NHS Blood and Transplant (2019) *The opt-out system*. Available at: www.organdonation.nhs.uk/supporting-my-decision/the-opt-out-system.

Organ Donation Taskforce (ODT) (2008a) *Organs for Transplants*. London: Department of Health.

Organ Donation Taskforce (ODT) (2008b) *The Potential Impact of an Opt out System for Organ Donation in the UK*. London: Department of Health.

Punch, J and Anderson, C (2012) Maastricht Type 2 Donors: unrealised opportunities. *American Journal of Transplantation*, 12(1): 9–10.

Reed, M and Lua, S (2013) Uncontrolled organ donation after circulatory death: potential donors in the emergency department. *Emergency Medical Journal*, 31(9): 741–44.

Reed, M and Lua, S (2015) The Royal Infirmary of Edinburgh Emergency Department Category 2 DCD Organ Donation Standard Operating Procedure. Unpublished.

Rodriguez-Arias, D et al. (2013) Casting Light and Doubt on Uncontrolled DCDD Protocols. *Hastings Centre Report* 43(1): 27.

Troug R (2010) Is it always wrong to perform futile CPR? *The New England Journal of Medicine*, 362(6): 477.

UK Donation Ethics Committee (2011) *An Ethical Framework for Controlled Donation After Circulatory Death*. London: Academy of Medical Royal Colleges.

Veatch R and Ross L (2015) *Transplantation Ethics,* 2nd Edn. Georgetown University Press.

Chapter 14	# Overview of Ethics and Legislation Surrounding Medicines

Andy Collen

Introduction

Medicines governance is one of the key aspects of paramedic practice. Paramedics are trusted in law to possess and administer a range of medicines for use in diverse and complex clinical presentations. The provision of medicines to patients in the urgent, emergency and critical care setting can be challenging – both legally and ethically. Patients may have very clear expectations about receiving certain types of medicines or they may have no knowledge or expectations, relying instead on the paramedic to guide their care entirely. The fact that paramedics, as a profession, are legally authorised to practise with the responsibility of using almost all legal mechanisms relating to medicines (depending on level and scope of practice, and employer authority) means that practice for paramedics involves the consideration of myriad factors associated with these different legislative and, of course, ethical drivers.

While it seems fundamental, paramedics sometimes get it wrong legally with medicines, and therefore the starting point must be to understand the mechanisms available to paramedics. By understanding the principles and limitations of each legal mechanism, paramedics can promote safe and effective care for patients, and approach their practice with confidence. Necessarily, the law which informs the use of medicines is specific and may appear restrictive, but the requirement to work within the law – despite the temptation to deviate based on patient need – is paramount.

This link between the legal, ethical and practical aspects of healthcare is particularly important when considering medicines. Broadly speaking, a medicine cannot be *ungiven* and therefore the approach taken must be considered and judicious – there is little room for the action-biased interventionist in a modern healthcare profession, and the desire to *do things to patients* must be challenged. Some medicines do need to be given and in the paramedic context need to be given quickly, but for the most part, there is always time to think and consider the medicines that are available.

In medicines-related practice, perhaps the most pertinent ethical consideration (beyond preventing harm) is the Kantian deontological principle which states that the subject (the patient) must never be *the means to an end* and must only ever be *the end in their own right* (Kant 1948). Each clinical encounter and its planned therapies must be based on the patient's needs alone. When this is considered holistically, along with the legislation and competence, the patient's safety will be promoted.

Paramedic Practice Guidance Relating to Medicines

The College of Paramedics, as the professional body for the paramedic profession, is required to publish practice guidance along with the other documents it publishes, such as curriculum and scope of practice guidance. Practice guidance is produced by all Allied Health Professions professional bodies and these documents form an important aspect of the role of these organisations (Allied Health Professions Federation 2018).

These documents are vital to ensure that paramedics have the information they need in practice, and these are specific to the profession. Legal mechanisms are not necessarily the same; for example, orthoptists are able to use exemptions to supply and administer listed medicines, whereas paramedics can only currently administer under exemption.

Practice guidance outlines the essential standards which need to be adhered to in practice in order to ensure that the legislation is upheld, patients are kept safe and paramedics can practise confidently and competently. The practice guidance supports and clarifies legislation, and works to remove ambiguity for clinicians in order to promote safe and confident practice (Royal Pharmaceutical Society 2016).

There are three main legal mechanisms available to paramedics:

- Exemptions
  - *Practice Guidance for Paramedics for the Administration of Medicines under Exemptions within the Human Medicines Regulations 2012* (College of Paramedics 2018a)
- Patient Group Directions
  - *Patient Group Directions* (National Institute for Health and Care Excellence (NICE) 2017)
- Supplementary and Independent Prescribing
  - *Practice Guidance for Paramedic Independent and Supplementary Prescribers* (College of Paramedics 2018b)

There are other mechanisms which do not necessarily have specific legislation assigned to them, but are also important to understand:

- Administration of prescribed medicines
- Patient Specific Directions
- Administration of non-prescription only medicine (POMs) using a protocol.

These additional methods of administering medicines are not covered in this book in detail, and any clinician (or associated professional) who is unsure should seek support from their employer's medicines governance team to ensure legal practice with authorisation to use these methods in practice. Many of the oral medicines cited in ambulance service practice guidance are General Sales List (GSL) or Pharmacy items (P), which can be administered under an organisational protocol. Practice guidance is not a legal mechanism, and paramedics should seek to ensure that where practice guidance serves as a protocol, the organisational policies clearly state this.

Exemptions

Legal exemptions are stated in the Human Medicines Regulations 2012 and allow stated groups to operate otherwise than in accordance with the Medicines Act 1968. The use of exemptions varies between the different groups in terms of what is exempt. For example, podiatrists can sell and/or supply courses of medicines under an exemption, but paramedics may only administer. Importantly, in the paramedic-specific exemption in Schedule 17 to the Human Medicines Regulations, the two following important statements appear:

> *The following prescription only medicines for parenteral administration.*
> *The administration shall be only for the immediate, necessary treatment of sick or injured persons and in the case of prescription only medicine containing Heparin Sodium shall be only for the purpose of cannula flushing.*
>
> (Human Medicines Regulations 2012)

These limitations in the legislation cannot be overlooked. Paramedics cannot use alternative routes for administration of the medicines listed (see Box 1) – for example, paracetamol cannot be given orally under this exemption and cannot be supplied either.

Importantly, most of the medicines listed in the list of exemptions are POMs and of these some are Controlled Drugs (CDs).

The Misuse of Drugs Regulations 2001, the wider legislation which prevents medicines from being accessed illegally and/or abused, provides additional statuses for CDs, organising them into classes and schedules. While it is broadly legal to possess any POM (or P/GSL), it is illegal to possess certain schedules of CDs and the exemptions which facilitate paramedic practice include a group authority to possess the controlled drugs listed (there is also specific allowance for certain CDs to be possessed using Patent Group Directions (PGDs) – see the section on PGDs below). The CD classes (A, B and C) relate only to their legal use (and risk of misuse) and have no relation to their therapeutic use. The schedule of CDs relates to the access and safe custody requirements for CDs in healthcare practice. For example, Schedule 1 CDs cannot be used in practice except where there is a special licence issued to use the medicine for clinical trials or other similar application. Schedules 2 and 3 are where strong opioids and benzodiazepines are scheduled (among other medicines). Weaker, oral opioids (such as codeine) appear in Schedules 4 and 5 (depending on whether it is mixed with another medicine, such as co-codamol). Safe custody of all medicines, but particularly CDs, is vital in promoting ethical, legal and safe practice.

CDs should be viewed with significant rigour, and the application of organisational policy and procedure must be observed in order to prevent loss and/or illicit use.

Legal exemptions list only the medicines which are exempt and do not include any information on dosing or other considerations. Therefore, any medicines used under an exemption must have an accompanying protocol, and clinicians using the medicines must be competent to use the medicines. There should be no presumption that because the medicine is listed as an exemption, this can or should be included in practice. Therefore, it should only be used where the clinician has been specifically trained to do so, or the employer has authorised administration, and an approved protocol can be followed.

Box 1   Schedule 17 Medicines – the Human Medicines Regulations 2012

- Diazepam 5 mg per ml emulsion for injection,
- Succinylated Modified Fluid Gelatin 4 per cent intravenous infusion,
- medicines containing the substance Ergometrine Maleate 500 mcg per ml with Oxytocin 5 iu per ml, but no other active ingredient,
- prescription only medicines containing one or more of the following substances, but no other active ingredient—
- Adrenaline Acid Tartrate,
- Adrenaline hydrochloride,
- Amiodarone,
- Anhydrous glucose,
- Benzylpenicillin,
- Compound Sodium Lactate Intravenous Infusion (Hartmann's Solution),
- Ergometrine Maleate,
- Furosemide,
- Glucose,
- Heparin Sodium,
- Lidocaine Hydrochloride,
- Metoclopramide,
- Morphine Sulphate,
- Nalbuphine Hydrochloride,
- Naloxone Hydrochloride,
- Ondansetron,
- Paracetamol,
- Reteplase,
- Sodium Chloride,
- Streptokinase,
- Tenecteplase.

There are two further schedules in the Human Medicines Regulations which provide exemptions that are relevant to paramedics: Part 3(9) of Schedule 17 (although this duplicates the medicines listed in Part 3(8) – the paramedic section) and Schedule 19. Schedule 19 lists a range of medicines that anyone can use in an emergency in order to save a life. This list duplicates many of the Schedule 17 medicines, but also includes antivenoms and antidotes. The medicines in Schedule 19 to the Human Medicines Regulations allow the following medicines to be administered by paramedics (see Box 2).

Box 2   Schedule 19 Medicines – the Human Medicines Regulations 2012

- Adrenaline 1:1000 up to 1 mg for intramuscular use in anaphylaxis
- Atropine sulphate and obidoxime chloride injection
- Atropine sulphate and pralidoxime chloride injection
- Atropine sulphate injection
- Atropine sulphate, pralidoxime mesilate and avizafone injection
- Chlorphenamine injection
- Dicobalt edetate injection
- Glucagon injection
- Glucose injection
- Hydrocortisone injection
- Naloxone hydrochloride
- Pralidoxime chloride injection
- Pralidoxime mesilate injection
- Promethazine hydrochloride injection
- Snake venom antiserum
- Sodium nitrite injection
- Sodium thiosulphate injection
- Sterile pralidoxime

Exemptions are a useful method for ensuring that paramedics can access medicines for immediate use in an emergency. Paramedics must ensure that they work within the confines of the law when using exemptions and must not deviate from the legislation. Practice guidance should always be followed to ensure that practice is safe and appropriate, and pitfalls are avoided, such as supplying medicines in error.

Patient Group Directions

PGDs became a legal entity in 2000, following recommendations made by Dr June Crown in her report from 1998. The Crown Report highlights gaps in care provision associated with access to medicines where prescribers are not available. PGDs are not in themselves a prescribing mechanism and are instead intended to treat patients who are not yet known to the clinician. Importantly, the word 'group' refers to cadres of patients who have a common disease process and can therefore be treated under a broad protocol – for example, patients over the age of 55 with a chest infection. Indication, dosage and routes of administration and/or method of supply are fixed in the protocol and allow only limited latitude to apply clinical judgement as to the suitability of patients to be treated using inclusion, exclusion and caution criteria.

PGDs are by their very nature prescriptive and cannot be deviated from. Clinicians who use PGDs must accept that their practice is confined by the limitations of the detail in the PGD. Again, the clue is in the name – Patient *Group* Direction – the group of patients at a population level who can be treated with antibiotics for a chest infection may not consider highly complex or unusual individual patient histories, underlying disease status, allergies or preferences. The temptation to deviate from the given conditions of a PGD in the interests of the patient must be avoided – if the patient does not belong to the *group* stated, they cannot be treated using the PGD and should be referred to a prescriber.

Patient Group Directions are legally defined in Schedule 16 to the Human Medicines Regulations 2012. This section of the legislation details the purpose and scope of the use of PGDs. Only specified healthcare professionals can use PGDs, including paramedics, and these clinicians can use the PGD to possess, administer and/or supply certain medicines. Most CDs are not able to be possessed under PGDs, and there are certain allowances for medicines such as ketamine and midazolam to be possessed under a PGD.

Unlike exemptions, which are universal, PGDs are organisationally specific and therefore care should be taken when working in different settings. The legal authority to use each PGD is derived from the signatories, and this cannot be done on behalf of another organisation (except where a specific contract or memorandum of understanding exists). This important consideration must be considered by paramedics who work across multiple organisations.

Another common error made with PGDs relates to the medicines provided as stock to supply to patients as a course of treatment. Medicines provided to be supplied as a course relate only to the PGD they are provided for. There is no mechanism for facilitating supply of medicines carried outside of a PGD, as even with a prescription from a doctor, the act of providing medicines in this way may be considered dispensing (particularly where the supply is repackaged), which can only be done by a pharmacist.

PGDs are extremely useful in paramedic practice settings and facilitate care for patients needing medicines to be supplied or administered. They are by their very nature restricted in their use, as suggested by the name of the mechanism, but this should detract from their utility. There is considerable guidance on PGDs available in legislation, and from the Medicines and Healthcare products Regulatory Agency (MHRA) and NICE, and developing an understanding of this mechanism provides an excellent opportunity to enhance practice and to start developing practice towards prescribing.

Independent and Supplementary Prescribing

Non-medical prescribing began in the early 1990s, following recommendations made in the Cumberledge Report (Department of Health and Social Security 1986), which suggested that limited formulary prescribing by district nurses would improve access to medicines for patients in the community. Prescribing was extended iteratively over the subsequent years, following the Crown Report written by Dr June Crown in 1989 (Department of Health 1989), and this paved the way for non-medical prescribing being extended beyond nursing and pharmacists. In 2013, physiotherapy and podiatry achieved independent prescribing responsibilities, and radiographers achieved supplementary prescribing. In 2017, dietetics achieved supplementary prescribing and paramedics achieved independent prescribing in 2018.

Definitions of Independent and Supplementary Prescribing

Independent Prescribing

Independent prescribing is prescribing by a practitioner who is responsible and accountable for the assessment of patients, and the planning of any treatments requiring the consideration of medicines. Prescribing practice may be seen in isolation as always inferring the addition of medicines to a patient's treatment plan, but in reality includes the decision to not prescribe and/or to de-prescribe, as well to prescribe.

Supplementary Prescribing

Supplementary prescribing is not a "lesser" mechanism compared to independent prescribing, and while its utility may be less relevant to paramedic practice, there are applications for its use. The basis of supplementary prescribing is that the patient has a Clinical Management Plan prepared by a medical independent prescriber in which a list of medicines is provided and against which a supplementary prescriber can prescribe. Supplementary prescribers must therefore have an existing relationship with their patients, and these patients must have a diagnosis and treatment plan in place.

Prescribing rarely involves the supply of medicines, and introduces the process of dispensing medicines in the presence of a prescription by a pharmacist, which has significant safety benefits. It is extremely important that paramedic prescribers understand the legal aspects of prescribing in their practice and how authority is derived, as well as the standards of practice which are required.

The law which informs the prescribing of medicines is the Medicines Act 1968. This piece of legislation is very well established and still provides the core tenets of medicines law in the UK. Subsequently, a range of regulations have been developed to help modernise care for patients, and the Human Medicines Regulations 2012 were developed to support the changes needed to facilitate non-medical medicines mechanisms. Specific to paramedics independent prescribing, the Human Medicines

Regulations were subject to an amendment in 2018 which authorised the changes made to the overarching regulations using the 'statutory instrument' (meaning that the change in the law did not require debate in the Houses of Parliament).

The responsibility for authorising prescribing for individuals falls to the professional regulator, which for paramedics is the Health and Care Professions Council (HCPC). The HCPC validates education programmes for prescribers and 'annotates' the registration of those individuals who fulfil the criteria as a prescriber. Annotation is in effect the legal authority for practical prescribing in practice and is subject to the usual HCPC scrutiny. Annotation, like core registration, may be subject to conditions in the event of a fitness to practice concern. Also, individuals with prescribing annotations must continue to fulfil the requirements of annotation for their prescribing practice and must voluntarily remove their annotation should their role change and cease to include prescribing.

Prescribing must be done in line with education, training, competency, supervision, audit and oversight. It requires a significant professional insight from the individual practitioner in order to ensure patient safety. Paramedic prescribing allows prescribing within the paramedic's scope of practice from the whole of the British National Formulary (BNF) (with the exception of CDs; cytotoxic drugs and specialist drugs).

The prescribing of controlled drugs is subject to additional safeguards, requiring additional changes to the Misuse of Drugs Regulations 2001, which may follow for paramedics after the changes to the Human Medicines Regulations 2012 are made. The Advisory Council on the Misuse of Drugs was formed to oversee the main piece of CD legislation – the Misuse of Drugs Act 1971 – and is responsible for considering changes to arrangements for controlled drugs in clinical care and other applications. Paramedics, common to all other allied health professional non-medical prescribers, have developed a short list of essential CDs which may be prescribed (subject to the changes in legislation required to permit this).

Independent and supplementary prescribing is the most significant medicines mechanism that any healthcare profession can practise using, and responsibility associated with prescribing requires well-developed professional insight. One of the most challenging situations for prescribers which differs from other mechanisms is the autonomy to decide what and when to prescribe rather than following a protocol. The constant tension between legal, ethical and practical considerations in practice applies to all medicines mechanisms open to paramedics, and highlights the trust in the profession by the establishment and patients.

Professional and Ethical Issues in Paramedics' Medicines Practice

As with many aspects of practice, professional fluency and a clear understanding of what is being asked of the clinician are of vital importance. For paramedics, the range of medicines, legal mechanisms, practice settings, and of course patient variety and demand, mean that navigating the legal and professional issues is extremely complex. When an ethical perspective is added – particularly where complex judgement is required by prescribers – the challenge becomes even more extreme.

There are additional considerations which should also be considered with all of the mechanisms within which paramedics practise using medicines, but particularly as our practice develops from exemptions, through PGDs and on to prescribing. These may be interpreted differently depending on the mechanism being used and are, to some degree, reliant upon the model of care and system being worked on, as well as the types of patients seen. Whilst there are many more concepts, the three brief definitions below demonstrate how medicines management is applicable across a range of ethical principles:

Rule-based (evidence-based) deontology

In its simplest form, deontology is the requirement to do the right thing (but does not assume doing things right). The duty-based effect of deontology may resonate closely with paramedics, particularly in the ambulance setting and when using medicines exemptions. Where protocols and clinical guidelines exist, this may infer a requirement towards action rather than a measured consideration to treat, and this may be justified by the linking of the *duty* aspects of rule-based care with the *doing-to* aspects.

Reductionism

Reductionism is the simplification of concepts; encompassing the most fundamental principles, it collectively accepts all of the detailed contributing aspects. For example, homeostasis could be considered a reductionist term as it *just happens* and you could (if you so desired) ignore all of the anatomical and physiological processes which exist to maintain it. As reductionism seeks to simplify concepts and actions, this may infer a blanket approach to tasks and dilemmas, leaving little room for further judgement. Again, this works well with protocol-based models of care and target-led cultures, but may grate with those practising at higher levels, including prescribers.

Positivism

Positivism is a principle which places that which is proven (or provable), or is established in law, over metaphysical concepts (such as belief systems), essentially placing the rules over morality. Giving every patient with chest pain aspirin, regardless of the lack of cardiac-sounding history or signs, is an example of this. It may be wrong from a rule-based perspective, but correct from a positivist standpoint – irrespective of the risks of giving aspirin without a true clinical indication. PGDs and exemptions-derived protocols are by their very nature positivist and leave no room for complex moral judgements in the presence of the patient being indicated for treatment.

Whilst the subject of biomedical ethics extends significantly beyond the scope of this chapter, these examples may form an ethical baseline for clinicians to consider their ethical standpoint on medicines. The world of ethics in healthcare is rich in literature and evidence, and is an area of expertise beyond the reach of most clinicians. Suffice to say that law and ethics exist closely, and in medicines-related practice they co-exist in a complex relationship.

> ### ✳ Case Study
>
> You are an advanced paramedic working in a walk-in centre. You are currently studying for your independent prescribing course, but, without supervision on this shift, are currently working under patient group directions.
>
> You see a 20-year-old female who is home from university, but has forgotten her medication for anxiety. She is normally prescribed diazepam 2mg three times a day and she shows you the emails she has exchanged with her own GP when she asked for advice. She has become jittery, paranoid and increasingly anxious, and, whilst she has tried to cope over the weekend without her medication, is really struggling.
>
> You have access to a PGD for Diazepam 2mg, but its only inclusion criterion is for muscular back pain or spasm. The nurse prescriber on the same shift has been quite unhelpful so far and you are keen to help this patient out, and so you document (falsely) that the patient has back pain and supply nine tablets of diazepam to her to ensure that she has sufficient tablets to get through the next few days before seeing her GP.
>
> - What ethical principles are at play here?
> - Has any legislation been breached by your actions?
> - What risks might your actions create for the patient?
> - What are the potential consequences for you as a clinician?
> - What could you have done differently to ensure that you upheld the ethical and legal imperatives?

Summary

Medicines legislation exists to ensure that the public are able to be treated safely and effectively with pharmaceutical therapeutic products, whilst controlling access to those medicines at a population level to guard against the risk of illicit use and criminality. Medicines legislation exists in two main groups: laws which control medicines for use on humans; and laws which control the possession of drugs and prevent misuse.

Paramedics may view legislation as restrictive and, in an age in which clinicians are ever more aware of the evidence base, may be tempted to practise outside legislative boundaries on the basis of promoting the best care for patients. Thinking back to the ethical principles discussed in Chapter 3, doing the right thing for patients (beneficence) and preventing harmful things from happening (non-maleficence) is crucial in promoting safe care. The notion of justice is important too; practising to, but not beyond, the limits of legal authority means that patients can be treated appropriately and without paramedics putting themselves in professional and/or legal jeopardy.

A clear understanding of the legislation is essential in roles which include the autonomous use of medicines – this is particularly so for the paramedic profession, which has the privilege of being able to practise using all of the main mechanisms (depending on their seniority and training) – exemptions, PGDs, prescribing – and the application of these mechanisms in practice requires consideration of the more appropriate mechanism to use, and not confusing or interchanging the approaches of each one. Primary education and ongoing professional development for paramedics should include a focus on medicines legislation and should also include other published guidance, such as Practice Guidance documents from professional bodies and other agencies (College of Paramedics 2018a, 2018b; Royal Pharmaceutical Society 2016).

Recommended Reading

Blaber, A, Morris, H, Collen, A (2018) *Independent Prescribing for Paramedics*. Bridgwater: Class Professional Publishing.

References

Allied Health Professions Federation (2018) *Outline Curriculum Framework for Education Programmes*. Available at: www.ahpf.org.uk/AHP_Prescribing_Programme_Information.htm.

British National Formulary (2018) *British National Formulary*. Available at: https://bnf.nice.org.uk.

College of Paramedics (2018a) *Practice Guidance for Paramedics for the Administration of Medicines under Exemptions within the Human Medicines Regulations 2012*. Available at: www.collegeofparamedics.co.uk/publications/independent-prescribing.

College of Paramedics (2018b) *Practice Guidance for Paramedic Independent and Supplementary Prescribers*. Available at: www.collegeofparamedics.co.uk/publications/independent-prescribing.

Department of Health and Social Security (1986) *Neighbourhood Nursing: A Focus for Care* (Cumberlege Report). London: HMSO.

Department of Health (1989) *Report of the Advisory Group on Nurse Prescribing* (Crown Report). London : Department of Health .

Department of Health (2012a) *Human Medicines Regulations (Schedule 16)*. Available at: www.legislation.gov.uk/uksi/2012/1916/schedule/16/made.

Department of Health (2012b) *Human Medicines Regulations (Schedule 17)*. Available at: www.legislation.gov.uk/uksi/2012/1916/schedule/17/made.

Department of Health (2012c) *Human Medicines Regulations (Schedule 19)* Available at: www.legislation.gov.uk/uksi/2012/1916/schedule/19/made.

Health and Care Professions Council (2013) *Standards for Prescribing*. Available at: www.hcpc-uk.org/resources/standards/standards-for-prescribing/.

Health and Care Professions Council (2016) *Standards of Conduct, Performance and Ethics*. Available at: www.hcpc-uk.org/standards/standards-of-conduct-performance-and-ethics/.

Kant, Immanuel (1948) [1785] *Grounding for the Metaphysics of Morals*. Cambridge, MA: Hackett.

Medicines and Healthcare products Regulatory Agency (MHRA) (2018) *MHRA*. Available at: www .gov.uk/government/organisations/medicines-and-healthcare-products-regulatory-agency.

National Institute for Health and Care Excellence (NICE) (2017) *Patient Group Directions*. Available at: www.nice.org.uk/guidance/mpg2/resources.

Royal Pharmaceutical Society (2016) *A Competency Framework for All Prescribers*. Available at: www.rpharms.com/resources/frameworks/prescribers-competency-framework.

UK Legislation

Human Medicines Regulations 2012

Medicines Act 1968

Misuse of Drugs Act 1971

Misuse of Drugs Regulations 2001

Chapter 15

Medical Research
John Renshaw

Introduction

In recent years, there has been a noticeable growth in the number of paramedics who are embarking on a career in research and are working within ambulance services research departments, clinical trials units and multi-disciplinary research collaborations (College of Paramedics 2017a; College of Paramedics 2017b; Paramedic PhD 2018). Previously, pre-hospital research was predominantly carried out by medical or nursing colleagues with a particular interest in pre-hospital care. However, more recently, paramedics have started to develop the knowledge, skills and experience to carry out original research in the pre-hospital setting. The welcome growth of research skills among the paramedic profession appears to have been facilitated by the introduction of research skills within pre-registration paramedic programmes and the integration of the research and development pathway within the College of Paramedics postgraduate career framework (see Figure 15.1) (College of Paramedics 2017c). Now that paramedics are able to pursue a career in research and make a more substantial contribution to multi-disciplinary research, the paramedic profession also needs to become familiar with the main legal, ethical and moral principles that support research that is ethically and scientifically sound (Health Research Authority 2017a; Paramedic PhD 2018).

The purpose of this chapter is to review the main ethical principles and considerations associated for paramedics undertaking research. It will focus upon the ethical standards, guidelines and applications that paramedic students, paramedics and early career researchers are most likely to encounter during the course of their studies, and will outline the process of submitting an ethics application to the Integrated Research Application System (IRAS).

What is Health Research?

The term 'health research' describes the process of systematically generating new, generalisable or transferable knowledge that can be used to either improve patient care, reduce uncertainties about treatment effectiveness or change how health services operate (Health Research Authority 2017b; National Institute for Health Research 2018). Research is fundamental to the development of health and social care as it helps to strengthen the evidence base to improve people's experience

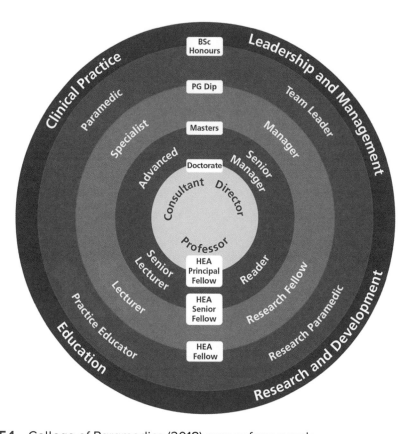

Figure 15.1   College of Paramedics (2018) career framework

of healthcare and provides unique access to some of the most cutting-edge treatments currently available (NHS England 2017, 2018). As one of the key providers of emergency and urgent care, paramedics use research during their patient assessment, physical examination and clinical decision making. Recently, ambulance paramedics have been more involved in research and have played an integral role in the recruitment of participants into large multi-centre clinical trials involving regional ambulance services (National Institute for Health Research 2017). As paramedics are gradually becoming more involved in research, they need to recognise their unconditional responsibility to carry out research to the highest ethical and professional standards mentioned in this chapter.

Research Ethics

The term 'research ethics' is commonly used to describe a set of moral principles that guide research from its initial planning stage through to its completion (British Psychological Society 2014). Whilst the main ethical principles of *autonomy*, *beneficence*, *justice* and *non-maleficence* are known to encompass most of the different moral issues that arise within healthcare (Gillon 1994), there are some additional ethical principles that are relevant to health research that require consideration. In the UK, the UK Policy Framework for Health and Social Care describes 15 key principles that act as a benchmark for good clinical practice in research, with a further four principles for interventional research design (Health Research Authority 2017a). Therefore, these ethical principles also set the standard expected for paramedic research.

Ethical Principles

The first ethical principle listed within the UK Policy Framework for Health and Social Care research is safety and the need to put the well-being of participants and researchers who are involved in the planning, collection or interpretation of the research before the interests of science (Health Research Authority 2017a). Subsequently, each member of the research team is required to possess the relevant education, training and skills to be able to conduct research that is scientifically and ethically sound (British Psychological Society 2014; Health Research Authority 2017c). Individuals who are less experienced can be deemed to be competent to perform tasks if they receive adequate supervision from a suitably qualified person (British Psychological Society 2014; Health Research Authority 2017c).

Research in health and social care should be designed to respect the rights, privacy, confidentiality, choice and well-being of everyone involved in research (Medical Research Council 2012). The information and data collected from participants needs to be handled correctly and stored safely to protect their confidentiality and right to privacy (Health Research Authority 2018a). Meanwhile, it is considered good practice for researchers to organise research projects within a documented protocol so that both researchers and participants can be clear about the design, objectives, methods of study, and the relevant legalities and ethical considerations associated with taking part in the study. The protocol should evidence the favourable ethical approval when it is expected or required and it should include information about research, such as its registration on the appropriate international research registries that help to prevent unnecessary duplication or waste (Health Research Authority 2018b; National Library of Medicine 2018). After all, research is thought to be a social process and researchers should appreciate their responsibility to discover new knowledge and information in the most effective and efficient way (British Psychological Society 2014).

Research participants must be afforded the respect and autonomy to decide whether or not they wish to take part in research. Therefore, participants should be provided with sufficient information in an understandable form to inform their choice to take part in the research, unless a university ethics committee agrees otherwise (British Psychological Society 2014; Health Research Authority 2018c). Participants must be able to easily differentiate between the proposed research and the standard care in order to be able to provide their informed and voluntary consent to take part (Health Research Authority 2018d). In addition, they should feel able to refuse or withdraw from the study without any reprisals and should be made fully aware of the benefits, potential risk of harm and inconvenience associated with the research. Accordingly, researchers also need to make adequate provision for indemnity and insurance to cover any potential liabilities that arise from being involved in the project (Health Research Authority 2017d). As registered healthcare professionals, paramedics who undertake research and do not comply with these fundamental ethical principles are likely to face legal challenges or the appropriate sanction from sponsors, employers and professional regulators (Health Research Authority 2017a).

Although the majority of these ethical principles are well established, one of the more recent principles to be factored into the planning and design stages is the need to build patient representation and public involvement throughout the research project (Health Research Authority 2018e). Patient representation is known to enhance the integrity, quality and improve the overall transparency of the research, and provides valuable experience of health and social care to promote a culture of openness, honesty and transparency between the researchers, participants and members of the public.

Finally, after the research has been gathered and interpreted, researchers have an obligation to accurately report and communicate their findings in a timely manner, regardless of whether their findings were positive or negative (Health Research Authority 2017a). The findings should also be made available to those who took part in the research, unless otherwise justified (Health Research Authority 2017a).

Important Regulations, Frameworks and Guidelines

The development of international standards for ethics in research is undoubtedly one of the most significant moments in the history of clinical research. These documents have subsequently enabled researchers from around the world to be able to collaborate on international projects with a shared understanding of the ethical principles, responsibilities and expectations associated with carrying out research involving human participants. Previously, researchers would have undertaken large international studies across many different countries, continents and cultures, and they would be challenged by the variations in the legal, ethical guidelines and local arrangements from each different country (World Medical Association (WMA) 2013). However, since the development of these overarching recommendations, researchers have a more streamlined understanding of ethical considerations in research, regardless of where the research is being undertaken (WMA 2013). Large international research collaborations are now relatively common in health and social care, and there appears to be a growing number of projects being carried out in the pre-hospital setting (Roberts et al. 2013). These examples demonstrate the possibility of undertaking international collaboration in the emergency and pre-hospital setting to the highest ethical and professional standard. In order to gain an overview of the relevant regulations, frameworks and guidelines for conducting research in the pre-hospital arena, paramedics need to

> **Pause for Thought**
>
> *Paramedics can find out more about international research within the International Guidelines for Health-Related Research Involving Humans publication from the Council for International Organizations of Medical Sciences (2016).*

have a basic understanding of the Nuremberg Code, the Declaration of Helsinki, the European Clinical Trials Directive, the Medicine for Human Use (Clinical Trials) Regulations 2004 and its amendments, and the UK Policy Framework for Health and Social Care (WMA 2013; Health Research Authority 2017a).

The Nuremberg Code (1947)

The Nuremberg Code is one of the most influential documents in the history of medical research ethics (Annas and Grodin 1992). This pivotal work stems from the Nuremberg trials in 1947, where Nazi doctors stood trial for conducting barbaric experiments on innocent victims and attempting to disguise their actions in the name of scientific research (Shuster 1997). The court's judgment in this trial subsequently contained 10 principles to protect everyone from harm during experimental and non-experimental research, which remain a powerful symbol for medical, nursing and allied health professionals involved in research. While the Nuremberg Code has never been fully adopted into law in the UK, it has undoubtedly become one of the most instrumental documents in the history of clinical research and many of its principles that serve to protect the rights of participants have subsequently been incorporated into international human rights agreements. As a starting point, it would be helpful for paramedics and student paramedics to have an awareness of the Nuremberg Code, each of the Code's 10 principles, and the history that led to its development. A summary of the 10 principles of the Nuremberg Code is given in Figure 15.2.

The Declaration of Helsinki (1964)

In 1964, the WMA announced the Declaration of Helsinki at the WMA General Assembly in Helsinki, Finland to provide ethical principles for medical research involving human subjects, or any of their material or data (WMA 2013). The original declaration was widely adopted by the international medical and scientific community; however, since then, there have been multiple amendments to the original version (WMA 2013). The Declaration of Helsinki has become the benchmark for ethical consideration for researchers who are conducting research involving human subjects that new proposals are compared to. In 2005, the Good Clinical Practice Directive included the recommendation for clinical trials to be conducted in accordance with the principles of the Declaration of Helsinki and this was transposed into UK law by the Medicines for Human Use (Clinical Trials) Regulations 2004 amended in 2006. Although it is not possible to discuss the Declaration of Helsinki in detail in this chapter, paramedics must review this important document, which makes specific recommendations in the following areas:

- general principles
- risks, burdens and benefits
- vulnerable groups and individuals
- scientific requirements and research protocols
- research ethics committees
- privacy and confidentiality

1. The voluntary consent of the human subject is absolutely essential. This means that the person involved should have legal capacity to give consent; should be so situated as to be able to exercise free power of choice, without the intervention of any element of force, fraud, deceit, duress, overreaching, or other ulterior form of constraint or coercion; and should have sufficient knowledge and comprehension of the elements of the subject matter involved as to enable him to make an understanding and enlightened decision. This latter element requires that before the acceptance of an affirmative decision by the experimental subject there should be made known to him the nature, duration, and purpose of the experiment; the method and means by which it is to be conducted; all inconveniences and hazards reasonably to be expected; and the effects upon his health or person which may possibly come from his participation in the experiment. The duty and responsibility for ascertaining the quality of the consent rests upon each individual who initiates, directs or engages in the experiment. It is a personal duty and responsibility which may not be delegated to another with impunity.

2. The experiment should be such as to yield fruitful results for the good of society, unprocurable by other methods or means of study, and not random and unnecessary in nature.

3. The experiment should be so designed and based on the results of animal experimentation and a knowledge of the natural history of the disease or other problem under study that the anticipated results will justify the performance of the experiment.

4. The experiment should be so conducted as to avoid all unnecessary physical and mental suffering and injury.

5. No experiment should be conducted where there is an a priori reason to believe that death or disabling injury will occur; except, perhaps, in those experiments where the experimental physicians also serve as subjects.

6. The degree of risk to be taken should never exceed that determined by the humanitarian importance of the problem to be solved by the experiment.

7. Proper preparations should be made, and adequate facilities provided to protect the experimental subject against even remote possibilities of injury, disability, or death.

8. The experiment should be conducted only by scientifically qualified persons. The highest degree of skill and care should be required through all stages of the experiment of those who conduct or engage in the experiment.

9. During the course of the experiment the human subject should be at liberty to bring the experiment to an end if he has reached the physical or mental state where continuation of the experiment seems to him to be impossible.

10. During the course of the experiment the scientist in charge must be prepared to terminate the experiment at any stage, if he has probable cause to believe, in the exercise of the good faith, superior skill, and careful judgment required of him, that a continuation of the experiment is likely to result in injury, disability, or death to the experimental subject.

Figure 15.2   The Nuremberg Code (as described in Shuster (1997))

- informed consent
- use of placebos
- post-trial provisions
- research, registration and publication and dissemination of results
- unproven interventions in clinical trials.

The Clinical Trials Directive (2001)

The European Commission (2018) describes a clinical trial as the scientifically controlled study of human participants in an attempt to establish, or verify, the effectiveness of investigational medicinal products (IMPs). In the EU, the conduct of clinical trials is governed by the Clinical Trials Directive (2001), which sets the minimum requirements for clinical trials in relation to:

- the protection of clinical trial subjects (Article 3)
- clinical trials on minors and incapacitated adults who are not able to give their legal consent (Articles 4 and 5)
- ethics committees and single opinion (Articles 6 and 7)
- detailed guidance (Article 8)
- commencement of a clinical trial, conduct of a clinical trial and the exchange of information (Articles 9, 10 and 11)
- suspension of the trial or infringements (Article 12)
- manufacture and import of investigational medicinal products and labelling (Article 13 and 14)
- verification of compliance of investigational medicinal products with good clinical and manufacturing practice (Article 15)
- notification of adverse events, serious adverse reaction and guidance concerning reports (Articles 16, 17 and 18)
- general provisions, application, entry into force and addresses (Articles 19, 22, 23 and 24).

As the Clinical Trials Directive is a legislative act, it subsequently requires each individual EU Member State to transfer the requirements and standards for clinical trials in Europe into its own domestic law. In the UK, it is the Medicines for Human Use (Clinical Trials) Regulations 2004 (as amended) that transpose this provision into UK law.

Notably, the European Commission has recently confirmed that the existing European Clinical Trials Directive will soon be replaced by the Clinical Trials Regulation, which hopes to streamline the rules for conducting clinical trials and the application procedures, improve the procedures in place for more thorough assessment, and strengthen the transparency of clinical trials data (European Commission 2018).

The Medicines for Human Use (Clinical Trials) Regulations 2004

The Medicines for Human Use (Clinical Trials) Regulations 2004 are the principal piece of legislation that transposes the EU Clinical Trial Directive into UK law and which subsequently sets the legal standard for clinical trials involving human participants. Although many of the original principles within the legislation are unchanged, there have been several different amendments over the past ten years that helped to correct errors in previous legislation, strengthen legislation surrounding an evolving area of research, implement new European directives into UK law, and regulate the collection of consent for minors and incapacitated adults in clinical trials . Consequently, paramedics should refer to the regulations *as amended* so that they include these compulsory changes and can understand the advancement of this legislation over time. Moreover, students, paramedics and early researchers should pay close attention to the statutory requirements for informed consent of participants in clinical trials of investigational medicinal products (CTIMPs), which also considers the challenge of collecting informed consent in an emergency situation (Health Research Authority 2014). A brief summary of some of the key definitions set out in Schedule 1 to the Medicines for Human Use (Clinical Trials) Regulations 2004 (as amended) is provided below.

Informed consent: research participants can only provide informed consent to take part in a clinical trial if they make their decision freely and are informed of the nature, significance, implications and risks of the trial (Health Research Authority 2014). In addition, they must either evidence their decision in writing, including the date, signature or mark by the person in order to indicate their consent, or if they are unable to provide this written consent then they can give their consent orally in the presence of a witness and recorded in writing (Health Research Authority 2014). This also applies to individuals providing informed consent as a person with parental responsibility or a legal representative on behalf of the trial subject (Health Research Authority 2014)

Capable adult: in order for capable adults to provide informed consent to take part in a clinical trial, they must have been interviewed by a member of the investigator's team so that they understand the objectives, risks and inconvenience involved in taking part. They must be made aware of their right to withdraw from the study at any time and must subsequently give their informed consent to take part. Participants who withdraw from a study by revoking their informed consent to take part do not have to provide a reason for their decision and this should not result in any reprisals. During the recruitment process, participants should be provided with a point of contact so that they are able to access further information about the trial if they so wish (Health Research Authority 2014). As a final point, it should be noted that if a participant has provided their informed consent to take part in a clinical trial and subsequently becomes unable to consent due to physical or mental incapacity, then their initial consent remains valid (Health Research Authority 2014)

Incapacitated adult: an incapacitated adult is someone who is unable to give their informed consent owing to a physical or mental incapacity. In clinical trials, informed consent can be provided on behalf of an incapacitated adult prior to the recruitment of the subject into the trial. The strength of this consent is arranged in a hierarchy of informed consent and this helps to identify who may be approached first to provide consent on someone else's behalf and in what condition. In England, Wales and Northern Ireland, personal legal representatives sit at the top of the hierarchy. Personal legal representatives must not be connected to the trial and they should be suitable to act as a legal representative owing to their relationship to the subject and be willing to do so (Health Research Authority 2014). In addition, researchers can approach professional legal representatives who also cannot be involved in the conduct of the trial. This is normally the doctor primarily responsible for the incapacitated person's medical care or a person nominated by a healthcare provider. That said, a professional legal representative should only be approached if there is no personal legal representative available (Health Research Authority 2014)

Emergency situations: in 2006, the Medicines for Human Use (Clinical Trials) Regulations 2004 were amended to make additional provision for incapacitated adults in emergency situations. This recognises that immediate treatment may need to be provided to an incapacitated adult as part of a clinical trial and there may be insufficient time to obtain written consent from a representative in this situation (Health Research Authority 2014). Therefore, the amendment allows for incapacitated adults to be entered into a clinical trial without prior consent being provided, as long as:

- the nature of the trial and the individual circumstances of the case mean that it is necessary to take urgent action for the purpose of the trial, but

- it is not practicable to obtain informed consent beforehand

- the treatment or action taken is carried out in accordance with a protocol approved by an ethics committee (Health Research Authority 2014).

In cases where an adult has been entered into a trial without giving informed consent during an emergency situation, researchers are expected to gain informed consent from either the subject or a legal representative after the emergency has passed and within a practicable timeframe (Health Research Authority 2014). If consent is withdrawn at these subsequent follow-up meetings, then patients should be removed from the clinical trial without reprisals (Health Research Authority 2014).

Helpfully, the Health Research Authority has created a short information note that condenses the requirements for informed consent within the amended clinical trials regulations, and it helps to clarify the position of gaining informed consent from minors or their legal representatives in an emergency (Health Research Authority 2014; Health Research Authority 2018c; Health Research Authority 2018d). However, as student paramedics are less likely to involve minors in their undergraduate or postgraduate research, it has been omitted from this chapter to maintain its focus. Nevertheless, it remains important legislation for research involving minors within the UK.

The Good Clinical Practice Directive (2005)

The Good Clinical Practice (GCP) Directive is an international ethical and quality standard that sets out the key principles and more detailed guidance for designing,

1. The rights, safety and well-being of the trial subjects shall prevail over the interest of science and society.

2. Each individual involved in conducting a clinical trial should be qualified by education, training and experience to perform his task.

3. Clinical trials shall be scientifically sound and guided by ethical principles in all their aspects.

4. The necessary procedures to secure the quality of every aspect of the trial shall be complied with.

5. The available non-clinical and clinical information on an investigational medicinal product shall be adequate to support the proposed clinical trial.

6. Clinical trials should be conducted in accordance with the principles of the Declaration of Helsinki.

7. The protocol shall provide for the definition of inclusion and exclusion of subjects participating in a clinical trial, monitoring and publication policy.

8. The investigator and sponsor shall consider all relevant guidance with respect to commencing and conducting a clinical trial.

9. All clinical information shall be recorded, handled and stored in such a way that it can be accurately reported, interpreted and verified, while the confidentiality of records of the trial subjects remains protected.

10. Before the trial is initiated, foreseeable risks and inconveniences have been weighted against the anticipated benefit for the individual subject and other presented and future patients. A trial should be initiated and continued only if anticipated benefits justify the risks.

11. The medical care given to, and medical decision made on behalf of, the subject shall always be the responsibility of an appropriately qualified doctor or, when appropriate, a qualified dentist.

12. A trial should be initiated only if an ethics committee and the licensing authority comes to the conclusion that the anticipated therapeutic benefits justify the risks and may be continued only if compliance with this requirement is permanently monitored.

13. The rights of each subject to physical and mental integrity, to privacy and to the protection of data concerning him in accordance with Data Protection Act 1998 are safeguarded.

14. Provision has been made for insurance or indemnity to cover liability of the investigator and sponsor which may arise in relation to the clinical trial.

Figure 15.3 Main principles listed within Articles 2, 3 and 5 of the GCP Directive (EC 2005/28) and The Medicines for Human Use (Clinical Trials) Amended Regulations (SI 2006/1928)

conducting, recording and reporting of clinical trials (Health Research Authority 2017a). It is important to distinguish that these standards are a supplement to the Clinical Trials Directive (2001) and have been transposed into law in the UK by the Medicines for Human Use (Clinical Trials) Amended Regulations 2006. While it is essential for paramedics to have a good knowledge of GCP involving the investigation of medicinal products, paramedics should be aware that these recommendations only apply to the clinical trials, and currently there is no legal requirement to conduct other types of research under these conditions. That being said, now that the paramedic profession is becoming increasingly involved in the recruitment of participants into clinical trials within the ambulance services, it seems sensible to review the main principles of good clinical practice. The main principles listed within Articles 2, 3 and 5 of the GCP Directive and the Medicines for Human Use (Clinical Trials) Amended Regulations are listed in Figure 15.3.

The UK Policy Framework for Health and Social Care Research

The UK policy framework for health and social care research provides a comprehensible summary of the principles of good clinical practice in the management of health and social care research (Health Research Authority 2017a). It sets out to reduce the amount of bureaucracy within research and tries to encourage researchers to utilise the resources that have been created to support the implementation of its key principles within health and social care research (Health Research Authority 2017a). Subsequently, this document provides a clear and relatively concise overview of the relevant legislation, ethical standards and international guidelines for ethical research, which may be particularly useful for student paramedics (Health Research Authority 2017a). It outlines various ethical principles, roles and responsibilities for researchers and healthcare professionals who are involved in research that includes patients, services users and their relatives or carers (Health Research Authority 2017a). Some of the main responsibilities that are discussed within the policy framework include the following:

- responsibility of individuals and organisations
- chief investigators
- research teams
- funders
- sponsors
- contract research organisations
- research sites
- regulators of professions
- other regulators
- employers
- health and social care providers (Health Research Authority 2017a).

Professional Guidelines

In the UK, there are multiple different research councils, professional societies and regulators that also publish their own guidance for researchers in a specific subject area or as part of a professional group. While most of the legislation, ethical principles and international guides mentioned in this chapter have focused upon clinical trials and research in the NHS, it is recognised that a large proportion of student paramedics and postgraduate students will not be undertaking clinical trials or research in health and social care. Therefore, it is important for prospective researchers to explore the various professional organisations, regulators and research associations in their area of research, as they may provide more relevant and specific guidance to their project. Some examples of different professional guidelines for ethics in research are listed below:

- The British Educational Research Association's *Ethical Guidelines for Educational Research: Fourth Edition* (2018).

- The British Psychological Society's *Code of Human Research Ethics* (2014).

- The Royal College of Nursing's *Research Ethics: RCN Guidance for Nurses* (Haigh et al. 2014).

- The General Medical Council's *Good Practice in Research and Consent to Research* (2013).

- The Medical Research Council's *MRC Ethics Guide: Medical Research Involving Children* (2004).

Applying for Ethical Approval

As soon as paramedics, and student paramedics, have become familiar with the legislation, guidelines and frameworks that support ethical research in emergency and pre-hospital care, they then need to develop their initial research proposal, identify which of the different approvals they require and subsequently submit their ethics application. Generally, paramedics will be able to determine what type of approval they will require, based upon what type of research is being undertaken, what method is being used, who is involved, where it takes place and whether the study involves the use of medicinal products or access to participants' personal information, for example. Henceforth, the remainder of this chapter will outline some of the most common approvals associated with undertaking research in the pre-hospital setting, namely, the NHS Health Research Authority and the NHS Research Ethics Committee (REC) (Health Research Authority 2018f). Notably, this section will describe the process for undertaking research involving adult patients in NHS organisations within England, as there appears to be some variation due to local policies in the application process between England, Wales, Northern Ireland and Scotland (Health Research Authority 2017a).

Research Proposals

Research proposals are one of the first documents that researchers are likely to work on during the initial planning and design stage of their research project. Proposals are thought to be particularly useful in terms of their ability to formalise an original research idea and expand it into a more coherent breakdown of the proposed study. As the proposal is developed, each member of the research team should be involved in the development, enhancement and subsequent review of the document over time, which will help researchers to refine their research questions and methods of study. While there are no firm templates for a research proposal as there are for more comprehensive research protocols, a research proposal will typically outline the background, aims, objectives, research questions, context to the research and method of study. For some time now, postgraduate university admissions teams have also used research proposals to help to assess an applicant's suitability for postgraduate study and to try to match them to an appropriate supervisor within the same field of work (University of Birmingham 2018).

Is My Project Classed as Research?

The Health Research Authority has consistently highlighted the need for researchers and managing organisations to be able to accurately determine whether their project is considered to be research, and whether it needs to be managed as such (Health Research Authority 2018e). The Health Research Authority has clarified that it is the managing organisation's responsibility to assess whether a project is classed as research, as this would then ultimately have to take on the role of research sponsor (Health Research Authority 2018e). However, paramedic researchers should appreciate the importance of this initial step as it can change how research projects are managed and will dictate what additional approvals and permissions are needed before the research can take place. Helpfully, the Health Research Authority has created an online decision tool entitled 'Is my study research?' in order to help prospective researchers decide whether or not their study meets the definition of research as described by the UK policy framework for health and social care research (Health Research Authority 2017a, 2018e). Therefore, it is advisable for paramedics to visit the online decision tool to determine whether their project is considered to be research, which is based upon the Research Ethics Service's more comprehensive table of research and non-research (Health Research Authority 2017a). The online decision tool considers at least three questions to determine whether a project is research and if researchers answer 'yes' to any of these questions, then the project is deemed to be research (Health Research Authority 2017a). The questions are as follows:

1. Are participants in your study randomised into different groups?

2. Are treatments, care or services allocated by randomisation?*

3. Is your study designed to produce generalisable or transferable findings?

(*Clinical Audit and Service Evaluation do not allocate treatments, care or services by randomisation according to protocol) (Health Research Authority 2017a).

University Ethics Committees

University ethics committees are structured to regulate the vast amount of research undertaken within higher education and to safeguard against research being undertaken that is undesirable, unethical or not well thought-out. Ethics committees work to preserve the integrity of research by ensuring that research applications comply with the aforementioned legal, ethical and professional requirements. Meanwhile, individual reviewers will assess each research application in order to determine whether researchers have accurately described the main ethical considerations within their area of study and have set out how they plan to overcome these issues within their application and research protocol. Reviewers are also required to ensure that each application complies with their university's policies, procedures and guidance for undertaking health research at university. Afterwards, and depending on the strength of the application, the ethics committee will either reject the application and explain its decision, or it will grant permission for the research to proceed within the specified timeframe based upon information provided. When ethical approval is awarded to a research project, the work will receive an individual reference number, which should be added to the research protocol to demonstrate ethical clearance and be published at a later date. However, it is important to recognise that university ethics committee approval may be insufficient for more research involving patients, service users or their relatives within the NHS, which will require external ethics approval from the NHS Health Research Authority Approval Service and/or the NHS REC. Lastly, paramedics should recognise that ethical approval is granted based upon the reviewer's assessment of the information provided; therefore, if there are any subsequent changes to this research project, the researcher would need to submit an amended application for additional review.

The Integrated Research Application System

The IRAS is a single-system online platform used to streamline the application process for research approvals within health and social care research (IRAS 2018). Previously, paramedics researchers were asked to submit their application across several different application platforms, which was time-consuming and generated a lot of unnecessary duplication.

However, the IRAS has subsequently enabled researchers to be able to create multiple different applications forms simultaneously based upon the information inputted by the researcher (IRAS 2018). As soon as paramedics have created an IRAS account and have started to input their details, the IRAS system will ask for a more detailed step-by-step breakdown of the proposed study and its core activities. Therefore, in order to increase the chance of being successful in their applications, paramedics are advised to seek the necessary guidance and preparation from their research supervisors beforehand. Completing an IRAS application form is one of the first initial steps in applying for either Health Research Authority or NHS REC approval (Health Research Authority 2018g). The various review bodies that are integrated in the IRAS are shown in Figure 15.4.

Research Protocols

The second step in applying for approval from either the Health Research Authority or the NHS REC involves preparing the necessary study documents and developing research protocols (Health Research Authority 2018h). Once paramedics have completed a research application on IRAS, they should then work to assemble their

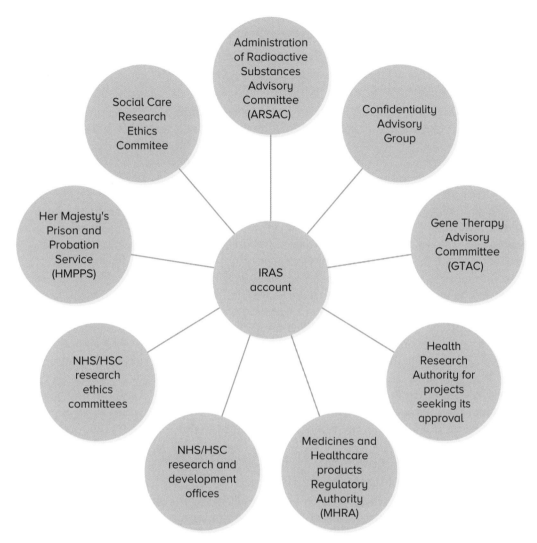

Figure 15.4 Summary of the approval bodies accessible through the IRAS (IRAS 2018)

participant information sheet, statement of activities, funding support and honorary contract information to support their application (Health Research Authority 2018h). As this chapter has already discussed, the GCP Directive makes it a requirement for researchers to describe their research design and justify the inclusion and exclusion criteria of their clinical trial within a research protocol. Research protocols are often compared to a project manual as they are known to organise research projects and provide a more comprehensive breakdown of each element for participants, researchers and the relevant review bodies (Health Research Authority 2017a). Consequently, they allow researchers to monitor the study's adherence to its approved study design and methodology. In recent years, it has become good practice to share and publish their completed research protocol, which can help to create an early scientific record of the proposed work and limit the wasteful duplication of research effort (Health Research Authority 2018b). Finally, paramedics are advised to utilise the

Health Research Authority's templates for clinical trials or qualitative research that have been designed to help researchers build their own research protocol with all the relevant elements included (Health Research Authority 2018b).

The Health Research Authority

The Health Research Authority aims to protect the interests of patients and members of the public by making sure that the research taking place within the health service is safe, legal and ethical (Health Research Authority 2018i). Its approval service currently provides an expert assessment of research governance and legal compliance for all project-based research applications within the NHS in England and Wales, alongside independent ethical opinion from the NHS REC (Health Research Authority 2018i; Health Research Authority 2018j). Before paramedics submit their Health Research Authority application, they should build their IRAS application, prepare the relevant research documents and use the Health Research Authority decision tool to confirm that their project is considered to be research. Afterwards, paramedics should then compare their project against the eligibility criteria in order to determine whether their project requires Health Research Authority approval, as illustrated in Figure 15.5. If their project does match the criteria for Health Research Authority approval, then paramedics will need contact the Central Booking Service to arrange an appointment with their nearest REC and submit their IRAS application on the same day (Health Research Authority 2018k). Research that does not meet the criteria for Health Research Authority approval but does involve a research tissue bank, a research database or is taking place in a non-NHS setting may require approval from the NHS REC and/or the Confidentiality Advisory Group (Health Research Authority 2018j). Most often, projects that are not classed as research do not require Health Research Authority or NHS REC approval.

The NHS Research Ethics Committee

The NHS REC is one of the core functions of the Health Research Authority and was set up to safeguard the rights, safety and well-being of participants taking part in research (Health Research Authority 2018j). In the UK, there are over 80 local RECs, which examine individual research applications in order to determine whether research is considered to be ethical, based upon all of the information provided (Health Research Authority 2018j). Thankfully, paramedics can now accurately determine whether their research project requires REC approval by using the Health Research Authority online decision tool entitled 'Do I need NHS REC approval?' and answering the questions as accurately as possible (Health Research Authority 2018g). It is likely that this online decision tool may be particularly helpful for paramedics who are undertaking research involving tissue banks, research databases or research taking place in a non-NHS setting, where REC approval may still be required (Health Research Authority 2018g). Meanwhile, paramedics who have identified that they require the opinion of the REC as part of their Health Research Authority approval may find this tool a little less relevant.

Once paramedics have created their electronic application via the IRAS and have contacted the Central Booking Service, they will be given an appointment at the

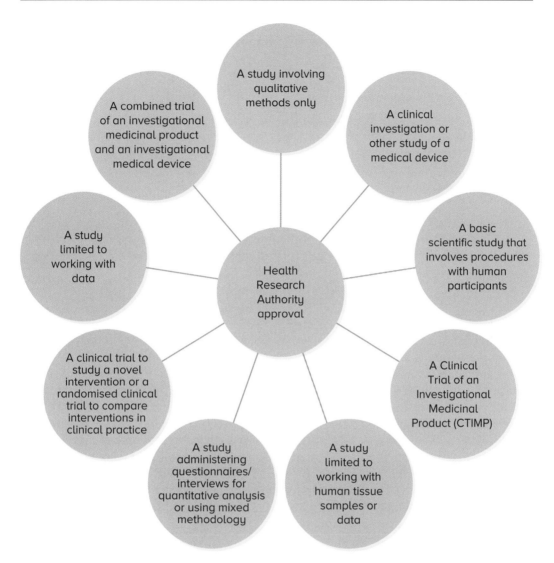

Figure 15.5 Diagram of the various types of research that require Health Research Authority approval (as listed on the Health Research Authority's website (Health Research Authority 2018))

nearest and most convenient REC meeting, depending on their type of study (Health Research Authority 2018k). Researchers are then required to submit their electronic IRAS application on the same day and await email confirmation of their appointment and confirmation that the submission is valid (Health Research Authority 2018k). In some cases, where their research is deemed to be particularly low risk on first assessment, paramedics may be entered into the proportionate review service (Health Research Authority 2018k). This service provides an accelerated review of research that has no significant issues and can elevate some of the pressure placed upon the larger RECs. Unlike a normal ethics committee meeting, a proportionate review may be reviewed via email, online conference calls or face-to-face meetings with smaller subcommittees (Health Research Authority 2018k). Research ethics committees aim to arrive at their decision within ten working days of the committee meeting. The four possible outcomes include:

- a favourable opinion to proceed
- a favourable opinion to proceed, but with conditions
- a provisional opinion
- an unfavourable opinion which doesn't not give permission (Health Research Authority 2018k).

Paramedics who receive a favourable opinion to commence with their research should note the Health Research Authority and REC approval number and share it with participants, sponsors, colleagues and members of the research team. They can then commence with their research project in the pre-hospital setting.

Summary

Over the past decade, there has been an exponential growth in the number of paramedics working in research or studying for postgraduate and doctorate programmes. Paramedics are now more likely to be involved in the recruitment of participants into studies within ambulance services, designing research proposals as part of an undergraduate programme or undertaking original research as part of a multi-disciplinary research team. Therefore, paramedics need to be familiar with the ethical considerations and challenges of conducting research in the pre-hospital setting. On a more practical level, they should know how to build an ethics application on the main digital platforms in order to be able to submit their application for review. Finally, while this chapter has provided a short overview of the ethical considerations in research, it cannot provide a comprehensive overview of such a broad topic, and so paramedics are encouraged to explore the attached recommended reading in more detail.

Paramedic research remains one of the most exciting and fast-moving areas of paramedic practice and, more excitingly, there is a lot of work to do. Go do it!

Recommended Reading

Davies, H et al. (2014) Guide to the design and review of emergency research when it is proposed that consent and consultation can be waived. *Emergency Medicine Journal*, 31: 794–95.

Guthrie, M (2014) Health and Care Professions Councils registrants participating in clinical trials. Available at: https://warwick.ac.uk/fac/sci/med/research/ctu/trials/critical/paramedic2/support/hcpc_registrants_participating_in_clinical_trials.pdf.

References

Annas, GJ and Grodin, MA (eds) (1992) *The Nazi Doctors and the Nuremberg Code: Human Rights in Human Experimentation.* New York: Oxford University Press.

British Educational Research Association (2018) *Ethical Guidelines for Educational Research: Fourth Edition*. Available at: www.bera.ac.uk/wp-content/uploads/2018/06/BERA-Ethical-Guidelines-for-Educational-Research_4thEdn_2018.pdf?noredirect=1.

British Psychological Society (2014) *Code of Human Research Ethics*. Available at: www.bps.org.uk/news-and-policy/bps-code-human-research-ethics-2nd-edition-2014.

College of Paramedics (2017a) *Paramedic Career Framework*. Available at: www.collegeofparamedics.co.uk/publications/digital-career-framework.

College of Paramedics (2017b) *Paramedic Curriculum Guidance*, 4th ed. Available at: www.collegeofparamedics.co.uk/publications/professional-standards.

College of Paramedics (2017c) *Post Graduate Curriculum Guidance*. Available at: www.collegeofparamedics.co.uk/publications/post-graduate-curriculum-guidance.

College of Paramedics (2018) *Post-Reg Career Framework*. Available at: www.collegeofparamedics.co.uk/publications/post-reg-career-framework.

Council for International Organizations of Medical Sciences (2016) *International Ethical Guidelines for Health-Related Research Involving Humans*. Available at: cioms.ch/shop/product/international-ethical-guidelines-for-health-related-research-involving-humans.

European Commission (2018) *Medicinal products: clinical trials*. Available at: https://ec.europa.eu/health/human-use/clinical-trials_en.

General Medical Council (2013) *Good Practice in Research and Consent to Research*. Available at: www.gmc-uk.org/-/media/documents/good-practice-in-research-and-consent-to-research_pdf-58834843.pdf.

Gillon, R (1994) Medical ethics: four principles plus attention to scope. *BMJ*, 309(6948): 184-8.

Haigh, C et al. (2014) *Research Ethics: RCN Guidance for Nurses*. Available at: www.yorksj.ac.uk/media/content-assets/research/documents/RCN-Research-ethics.pdf.

Health Research Authority (2014) *Medicines for Human Use (Clinical Trials Regulations) (2014): informed consent in clinical trials*. Available at: www.hra.nhs.uk/documents/294/informed-consent-in-ctimps.pdf.

Health Research Authority (2017a) *UK Policy Framework for Health and Social Care Research*. Available at: www.hra.nhs.uk/planning-and-improving-research/policies-standards-legislation/uk-policy-framework-health-social-care-research.

Health Research Authority (2017b) *Defining research table*. Available at: www.hra-decisiontools.org.uk/research/docs/DefiningResearchTable_Oct2017-1.pdf.

Health Research Authority (2017c) *Research: before you apply for approval*. Available at: www.hra.nhs.uk/research-community/before-you-apply/protocol.

Health Research Authority (2018a) *Confidentiality Advisory Group*. Available at: www.hra.nhs.uk/approvals-amendments/what-approvals-do-i-need/confidentiality-advisory-group.

Health Research Authority (2018b) *Protocol*. Available at: www.hra.nhs.uk/planning-and-improving-research/research-planning/protocol.

Health Research Authority (2018c) *Informing participants and seeking consent*. Available at: www.hra.nhs.uk/planning-and-improving-research/best-practice/informing-participants-and-seeking-consent.

Health Research Authority (2018d) *Consent and participant information guidance*. Available at: www.hra-decisiontools.org.uk/consent/principles-ALC-EnglandandWales.html.

Health Research Authority (2018e) *Is my study research?* Available at: www.hra-decisiontools.org.uk/research.

Health Research Authority (2018f) *What approvals and decisions do I need?* Available at: www.hra.nhs.uk/approvals-amendments/what-approvals-do-i-need.

Health Research Authority (2018g) *Do I need NHS REC approval?* Available at: www.hra-decisiontools.org.uk/ethics.

Health Research Authority (2018h) *Applying to a Research Ethics Committee*. Available at: www.hra .nhs.uk/approvals-amendments/what-approvals-do-i-need/research-ethics-committee-review/ applying-research-ethics-committee.

Health Research Authority (2018i) *HRA approval*. Available at: www.hra.nhs.uk/ approvals-amendments/what-approvals-do-i-need/hra-approval.

Health Research Authority (2018j) *Research Ethics Committee Review*. Available at: www.hra .nhs.uk/approvals-amendments/what-approvals-do-i-need/research-ethics-committee-review/

Health Research Authority (2018k) *Central Booking Service*. Available at: www.hra.nhs.uk/about-us/ committees-and-services/central-booking-service.

Integrated Research Application System (IRAS) (2017) *A step by step guide to using IRAS to apply to conduct research in or through the NHS/HSC*. Available at: www.myresearchproject.org .uk/help/hlpnhshscr.aspx.

Integrated Research Application System (IRAS) (2018) *Homepage*. Available at: www .myresearchproject.org.uk/SignIn.aspx.

Medical Research Council (2004) *MRC Ethics Guide: Medical Research Involving Children*. Available at: mrc.ukri.org/documents/pdf/medical-research-involving-children.

Medical Research Council (2012) *Good Research Practice: Principles and Guidelines*. Available at: mrc.ukri.org/publications/browse/good-research-practice-principles-and-guidelines.

Montgomery, J (2003) *Healthcare Law*, 2nd ed. Oxford: Oxford University Press.

National Institute for Health Research (2017) *National Institute for Health Research Activity League Table 2016–2017*. Available at: www.nihr.ac.uk/research-and-impact/nhs-research-performance/ league-tables/older-league-tables.htm

National Institute for Health Research (2018) *Why research matters: what is research?* Available at: www.nihr.ac.uk/patients-and-public/why-join-in/why-research-matters.htm.

National Library of Medicine (2018) *ClinicalTrials.gov*. Available at: https://clinicaltrials.gov/ct2/home

NHS England (2017) *NHS England Research Plan*. Available at: www.england.nhs.uk/publication/ nhs-england-research-plan.

NHS England (2018) *Supporting Commissioners: Research*. Available at: www.england.nhs .uk/commissioning/supporting-commissioners/research.

Paramedic PhD (2018) *Registers: paramedic register*. Available at: www.paramedicphd.com.

Roberts, I et al. (2013) The Crash-2 trial: a randomised controlled trial and economic evaluation of the effects of tranexamic acid on death, vascular occlusive events and transfusion requirement in bleeding trauma patients. *Health Technology Assessment*, 17(10): 1–79.

Shuster, E (1997) Fifty years later: the significance of the Nuremberg Code. *New England Journal of Medicine*, 332(20): 1436–40.

University of Birmingham (2018) *How to write a research proposal*. Available at: www .birmingham.ac.uk/schools/law/courses/research/research-proposal.aspx.

World Medical Association (WMA) (2013) *WMA Declaration of Helsinki – Ethical Principles for Medical Research Involving Human Participants*. Available at: www.wma.net/policies-post/ wma-declaration-of-helsinki-ethical-principles-for-medical-research-involving-human-subjects.

UK Legislation

Medicine for Human Use (Clinical Trials) Regulations 2004 (SI 2004/103)

Medicines for Human Use (Clinical Trials) Amended Regulations (SI 2006/1928)

Medicines for Human Use (Clinical Trials) Amended Regulations (SI 2006/2986)

Medicines for Human Use (Clinical Trials) Amended Regulations (SI 2008/941)

EU Directives

Clinical Trials Regulation (EU 536/2014)

European Clinical Trials Directive (2001/20/EC)

Good Clinical Practice Directive (2005/28/ECs)

Index